FROM

TRAGEDY

TO

TRIUMPH

THE STORY OF JOHN TARTAGLIO

John Tartaglio
Andrew Chapin

No Limits books may be purchased for educational, business, or sales promotional use. For information address No Limits Publishing– Attention: From Tragedy To Triumph, 1000 North Street, Milford, CT 06461

No Limits Publishing

FIRST EDITION

Cover designed by Nick Abriola.

John Tartaglio is available to speak at your live event. For more information or to book an event, visit www.johntartaglio.com or call (916) 237-7325.

ISBN: 978-0-9912592-1-2
ISBN-10: 0991259211

PREFACE

I want you to imagine living a more confident life. I want you to imagine living a more fulfilling and happy life. I want you to imagine living a life where you set goals and achieve results that go beyond even your own wildest expectations.

In the business world, one way that a company drives performance and change is through the congruence model. The simple idea is that when a company sets its goals, its results are based off of meeting the mission of the organization. To help it meet these goals, it aligns each aspect of the organization to reinforce and support them.

In the same way, the model I have developed says that we need to set our goals based on what we value, that is what has the most meaning to us. In order to meet these goals, we must align each aspect of our lives to reinforce and support what our goals are.

This is a dynamic model where our experiences continue to shape who we are and what we value. In independent research I conducted, I found data that was statistically significant to support the model. The result is that when executed, not only do we meet our goals, but we also live more fulfilling, happy, and confident lives.[1]

Besides the quantitative data, I'm living proof. I woke up with no legs and my world changed; I didn't know how the rest of my life would be. As time went on, I became more independent. In the same way, I used competition as a way to overcome my disability. Event after event that I completed, I saw that I could do more.

---

[1] There was a positive correlation (R-value .65 or greater) among how fulfilled people were with each aspect of their lives, how each aspect aligned with what they valued, and how fulfilled, happy, and confident they were. Stepwise regression models resulted in the most significant variable (P-value less than .05), how well each aspect aligned to fit what subjects valued most, which affected people's resulting fulfillment, happiness, and confidence.

At various points throughout *From Tragedy to Triumph*, I reflect on what I have learned from my experiences in the form of journal entries. My hope is that this will help you live a better life on your own terms.

Value Based Growth Model

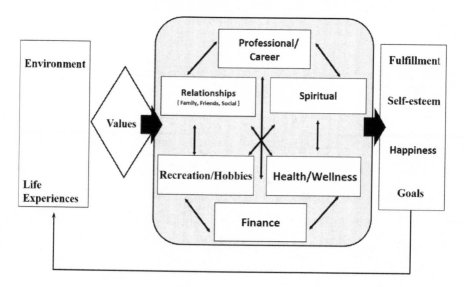

PROLOGUE

I literally remember thinking to myself, "This is going to be the day that I die."

My legs were an alarm, pulsating pain throughout my lower limbs. Sweat streamed down my face. Feverish, then freezing, I shivered.

Hours passed in that hospital bed, incapacitated by the unidentified agony that wracked my body. With no other solution, the doctors pumped me full of morphine until I passed out. On the cusp of consciousness, my thoughts were grave. *What is happening to me? What is wrong? Where have the doctors gone?* I was in and out, like a wave washing against the shore and the tide pulling it out again.

Caught in a riptide-like fury, there was a frenzy of activity going on around me. And there I was, helpless, being poked and prodded. Everything was happening so quickly now that reality seemed to blur; I was merely a bystander, and my world was unfolding before me like I was underwater with no way of reaching the surface.

When I awoke again, I was on a stretcher surrounded by my family. Their eyes were watery; some were even crying. The mood was as somber as that at a wake. Were they mourning me? No, I was still very much alive, but I could not dismiss the thought that pervaded my mind: *This is going to be the day that I die.*

I knew the situation wasn't good, but how bad it was no one knew. Not me, not my parents, not my doctors. I was caught in the current of an unknown ailment, fighting desperately to make my way back. *Tell me something, anything, so I can assure all of these concerned spectators that there's nothing to see here and they can all go home.*

There was an acute urgency building up inside of me despite the anesthetizing effects of all the medication. I wanted to burst out of bed, run through the hospital corridors, and proclaim myself cured. But I wasn't. My legs were the size of waterlogged tree trunks. When I touched them, I heard a crackling sound, like popcorn sizzling on the stove. I wasn't at all.

I was pulled back under by the tide of uncertainty. When I would wake again I was not sure. If I would wake again was not a guarantee. From that moment on, nothing in my life was a guarantee.

FROM

TRAGEDY

TO

TRIUMPH

THE STORY OF JOHN TARTAGLIO

John Tartaglio
Andrew Chapin

1

Growing up, my interests were as simple and fulfilling as any other kid's: playing sports, having fun, and doing well in school. Girls did not matter yet. Most of my classmates were friendly, not yet separated by the superficial differences that divide with age—that was until it came time for the gym class fitness test.

I was in eighth grade and at that awkward stage of physical development where my body was as disproportionate as a funhouse mirror. Now, I was being compared to my peers—they with their toned muscles and unending energy and I with my flabby physique and sluggish pace. Trapped in my chubby adolescence, I could barely do a push-up before my back collapsed under my own weight. And the mile run was a punch to the stomach, a shot to the gut that branded me indelibly as weak.

Secretly, I was ashamed. I hated it all—the test, my showing, my body—everything that made me stand out as the fat kid. I was uncomfortable with who I was, but I could not reveal my true feelings. Guys were not supposed to worry about their weight.

So I began to compensate for it like it was a physical deficiency. I would hide my hurt by being the funny guy, the brunt of his own jokes and others' as well. My jovial, personable exterior was a cover for my self-consciousness. Even with my closest friends, my weight would somehow become the focal point of their jokes. I laughed at my weight, they laughed at my weight, EVERYONE laughed at my weight.

After a while, I was tired of laughing at myself. I did not want that oversized shadow following me around any longer. I was going into high school, and it was time for a change.

What started out as a focus on my general outward appearance evolved into an overall change in my lifestyle. After reading Bill Phillips's *Body for Life*, I stopped waiting around for a growth spurt and actively took control of my health. Gone were the ravenous meals of the past, replaced with balanced meals and regular exercise. I became addicted to the routine. It was no longer about how I looked. It was about how I lived.

Early on in high school, I played football and baseball, yet my true passion was not for the love of the game but rather the physical challenge of it. Injuries eventually took me off the field, but I knew that I did not need sports to maintain my personal health. The only competition I was in was with myself.

Biology became my new game, and I found an ally in my teacher. He, an avid cyclist, gave me a perspective on life that guided me into adulthood.

"Being quietly confident will get you far in life," he said. I would not boast, nor brag, nor degrade others. I would simply be me, working to achieve my ambitions despite doubts and detractions. And I would.

****

Sitting in a Kaplan SAT review class on a steamy July day, I felt like I was in the freezer. A cold sweat hung from my brow as I tried to control my chomping teeth and complete a practice test. After each question, I seemed to feel worse. As I handed in the test, I knew that I had a fever, but I headed to work anyway.

I had barely made it through the restaurant doors before my coworkers agreed that I needed to be sent home. All I wanted was my bed, but it was like I was in a sauna. As I poured sweat through layers and layers of bed sheets, my fever resisted rest and stubbornly boiled to 103 degrees before my mother took me to the hospital.

Charts were examined, tests were ordered, blood was extracted, results were examined, more tests were ordered, and close conversations were had. Yet there were no answers. My body that I had so meticulously taken care of over the years was waging a civil war against me.

In the hospital bed with my mother by my side, I waited hours before the doctors' shaking heads and noncommittal expressions answered my question. All of the tests came back negative.

"Can't you give him an antibiotic?" my frustrated mother pleaded with the doctor.

Again, there were no answers. "No. It's just a virus." His voice had neither promise nor condemnation. It was neutral, the kind that becomes conditioned from years of devastation. I was discharged from the hospital with instructions of "bed rest and aspirin" that I begrudgingly had to accept. Still, there was no diagnosis.

For a week, I swam through my sheets restlessly tortured by my schizophrenic temperature. It would subside, giving me reason to believe I was getting better. Then, like a game of keep-away, my fever would spike and snatch away any hope I had.

No matter what medicine I took or how much rest I got, I felt like I was seventeen going on seventy. It was the summer going into senior year, and my friends were out being young while I was bedridden. I just wanted to be a kid again.

After all of the tests, all of the negative results, and all of the unknowns, there was finally some clarity to my situation. I had mononucleosis, or mono, my primary care physician explained to me. He prescribed me another month of rest and restricted activities. That meant no work, no exercise, no friends, no fun. But at least I knew what I was dealing with.

As the world passed by my window, I slowly began to feel like myself again. *It's almost over.* My body, which had held me captive for over a month, was finally exonerating me. I couldn't wait to be a teenager again.

2

My teeth were chattering like Chiclets in a shaking box. It was Sunday, August 22, 2004, at about 7:00 a.m. I struggled to get up. *Could it be growing pains?* Arched with ache, I finally lumbered out of bed on my way to the bathroom. It took me fifteen minutes to get to a door that was a mere fifteen feet away. *What was going on?* I was supposed to be getting better, not worse.

"Mom," I whispered into my parents' room, trying not to wake my father. "I think something's wrong. My legs are really killing me." We tried every household remedy, but no amount of Icy Hot could ease my pain.

****

Just getting to my feet had become an excruciatingly difficult task. As I staggered into the doctor's office, I decided that I would rather run a marathon on a broken leg than feel this sensation again.

With childlike stubbornness, the pain refused to subside. When my doctor finally arrived, I was disabled. Having lost all function in my legs, I described my symptoms to him. A urine test was ordered, but he was not compassionate to my situation. When I asked him if someone could take me to the bathroom, he snidely replied, "Well, how do you expect to get back home if you can't walk?" With no help from him or his assistants, my mother had to wheel me to the bathroom to complete the test because I could not stand.

The test showed that I had a condition called myositis. My body was breaking down muscle and expelling it as a waste product in the form of protein in my urine. It sounded much worse than it actually was, the doctor assured us. This was no cause for alarm, he said, but with the slight potential that my kidneys could begin to shut down, I would have to stay overnight at Yale New Haven Hospital for further tests.

****

Sweat streamed down my face; I was feverish yet freezing at the same time. As I slipped in and out of consciousness, doctors and nurses frequently asked me, on a scale of one to ten, what was my pain level.

"Nine," I moaned. The morphine dripped. Hours passed. The question was asked again. "Nine." My teeth gnashed. *Still nine.* Fingers clenched the sheets. "Nine!" The morphine trickled. *Always nine.* My eyes fell. I was out.

"Mom," I muttered, my subconscious breaking through my slumber. "My legs are killing me. Get these off me!" When I opened my eyes, she was next to me and I was still in a hospital bed. *This nightmare is actually happening.* I was very much conscious by this point, and my arm looked like it was suffocating.

"Please tell me what is going on," my mother pleaded with the nurse. "Why is my son's arm turning blue?"

A female doctor rushed in. "Broad spectrum antibiotics!" she instinctively yelled. "We need to move!"

****

"Mrs. Tartaglio," the doctor said, "I have some very bad news. Your son is dying..."

Before she could finish her sentence, one she had probably pronounced so many times and would so many times more, my mother broke down.

"You're WRONG!" she screamed. "The test confirmed myositis. The test..." crying out again, "...confirmed myositis!" She repeated this over and over again, trying to convince herself against a reality she refused to accept.

"Your son looks too damn good to be so sick, but he is," the doctor said as she tried to console my mother in her cold, dispassionate tone. "He is experiencing necrotizing fasciitis, a flesh-eating bacteria. In cases like this, the survival rate is around twenty percent. I'm sorry, I know this must be hard, but we need to act quickly if he has any chance."

Even with my sister Jennifer by her side, my mother was in a frenzy of inconsolable emotion. "I believe in miracles!" she wailed. It was as if she was the one fighting for her life. "He will survive."

****

Touching my legs, I asked my father, "Do you hear that crackling? It sounds like popcorn."

My parents told me that I was about to go in for a "minor exploratory surgery," but I knew that whatever was going on was far worse than a precautionary overnight hospitalization. My entire family, including aunts and uncles, surrounded me. *If this surgery is so minor, why are they all looking over me like I'm already dead?* Before I went, I called my girlfriend; she wasn't home. I never thought I would see her again.

****

Cutting a deep, longitudinal slit into my thigh, the doctors tried to explore the depth of my spreading infection. After the fasciatomy, my situation became that much more dire. The crackling sound in my legs was really the movement of gas gangrene trapped underneath my skin, inside of my legs. This gas was the result of a bacterial infection that caused severe muscle tissue death.

While the doctors searched for a remedy to my illness, a Lifestar helicopter shuttled me over to Norwalk Hospital, a decision my parents made based on its proximity to our house, and, most importantly, because I was running out of time. I needed a hyperbaric chamber, a vessel that

7

provides only pure oxygen, in order to fight the anaerobic bacteria. Norwalk Hospital provided this accommodation.

Word was traveling fast; prayer chains were constructed in many homes around the town. My friends hurried to the hospital to be by my side, friends who I had just seen days before. I looked like the same healthy John they had always known. Now, no one was sure if I would make it through the night.

****

A special surgeon, Dr. Crum, was called in. He had experience dealing with this kind of bacterial infection.

"Do whatever it takes to keep that boy alive," my parents said.

Hours before, they were under the impression that everything would be fine, that it was not as bad as was first thought, and that the hyperbaric chamber was the cure-all remedy. Now, the only chance that I had was for the doctors to amputate the infected areas of my body.

At around 2:00 a.m., approximately twenty members of my close family and friends gathered. Out of surgery, Dr. Crum informed my mother, "We had to take part of your son's left bicep, and we had to amputate his legs." Deep down, my parents had anticipated this ultimate outcome, and the doctor did not sugarcoat it. "The next forty-eight hours are critical to John's survival."

"What are you saying, Doctor?" My father, doubled over like a punch to the stomach, gasped for air. "He was perfectly healthy, and now he is going to die?" These were terms that neither of my parents would accept, but reality was cold and unforgiving.

The bacteria, which had started in my thighs, were moving upward. My surgeons had to stop it from spreading; however, they were unsure how far up they would have to amputate in order to stop it. The only option I had was to undergo debridement surgeries where the

8

surgeons identified infected muscle tissue and then proceeded to scrape and cut it away.

Over the course of five days, I endured five major surgeries and four sessions in the hyperbaric chamber. The doctors tried to take as little of my limbs as possible, but they were at the mercy of the bacteria. They had no choice but to remove both of my legs, including my femurs. My parents were told that I would never walk again.

Now, all my doctors could do was hope. They were unsure if the bacteria had affected my vital organs, brain functions, or my ability to communicate. However, Crum was able to prevent the bacteria from spreading beyond my legs and into my reproductive organs and digestive tract.

****

Waking up inside of the hyperbaric chamber, my memories were as vague as undeveloped film. I looked around tentatively. My left arm was strapped to a board. I had tubes everywhere. In my arms. In my neck. In my mouth. I wanted them out. I wanted out! I tried to scream, but I could not.

As strong as my parents were for me, they could not bring themselves to tell me what had happened. Instead, I heard my nurse's voice. "In order to save your life, the doctors had to amputate your legs and left bicep."

She continued to speak, but her words became foreign, indiscernible over the emotions that barreled and crashed against my insides.

I had done nothing wrong. Why did I deserve such a destitute fate? How would I be able to do what other kids my age did? Would I ever be able to live a normal life? What was a normal life for someone like me?

Then there were no thoughts, just my blank face and the tears running down it. I was as numb as my nonexistent limbs. I closed my eyes. This nightmare could wait.

So many people ask me what that moment was like when I first realized what had happened. For me to sit here and write that I was not devastated, upset, and angry would just be a lie. I woke up one day to find out that I no longer had legs after seventeen years, and I knew my life would never be the same. It was the silent times at night while my mother or my father and I were trying to go to sleep that were the worst. I could not help but think about anything besides what had happened and what my limitations were going to be. There I was upset, lying in a hospital bed that turned me because I could not turn myself, thinking about how different my life was going to be with no clue how it would go.

When people were around, I had an escape, a way to socialize as if nothing had changed. This was my way of coping, using a stone-cold exterior, acting as if nothing had ever happened. Some thought this was courageous, but if I did not stay strong for my family and my friends, they would have to go through much more painful times. And that would just not be fair.

Their support allowed me to continue on and ultimately changed my way of thinking; they were a constant reminder of all that I still had to live for, so my perspective shifted away from the pessimism and negativity toward a more glass-half-full approach.

It is not easy for people to understand how I could stay positive, but the alternative is a dead end. Regardless of how I felt or what I did, I knew I could not change what had happened to me. If I spent too much time contemplating "why me," the experience would dictate my life and I would never have been able to grow to become the person I am today. I was lucky to be alive, and I reminded myself of that every day.

Realistically, there is no surefire way for anyone going through troubling times to cope, but what I do know is that the upbeat attitude that I tried my best to exude helped me tremendously. Sometimes when people deal with adversity, they get stuck in a negative moment; it consumes their thoughts and paralyzes them from moving forward. It is important to take it step by step and remember that you have the opportunity to do something positive for yourself and for others on a daily basis. We all have the power to be positive influences.

3

Hastily scribbled on the whiteboard was the following: SHUT UP! I'M REALLY TIRED!

My family laughed at my cranky reaction to the incessant questions my mother was asking me. It was simple and to the point, but I did not have any other choice. With the breathing tube still protruding from my mouth, I had to rely on a dry-erase board in order to communicate.

To aid the nurses and myself, a trapeze was set up above the hospital bed. While I was still physically weak from my traumatic experience, the trapeze gave me hope that becoming independent was possible. It allowed me to pull myself up when I needed to be changed or when my sheets needed to be cleaned. My life was certainly going to be different, but I refused to lose my ability to function, my ability to *do* in society.

During my hyperbaric chamber sessions, I encountered a particular nurse who took a motherly watch over me. She would try and talk to me about what I did not remember. Her kindhearted intentions were not lost on me. She allowed me to shave my face on my own. It was an act so miniscule in the scope of everyday life that it would go unnoticed almost anywhere else. In my situation, however, she had given me dignity and allowed me to keep some of my independence.

As the doctors continued to test me like a sample, the facts of my illness were still vague. What they knew was that I had been stricken with an extremely rare bacterial infection, so rare in fact that I was one of only thirty-five people in medical history to contract it. While previous patients who had the infection were much older and their immune systems were vulnerable due to cancer, chemotherapy treatments, and AIDS, there had never been a case like mine.

Outside of the statistics, they could not determine what had caused the bacterial infection; all they could report was that my immune system had been compromised and I had contracted clostridium septicum along with pyomyositis, the rare duo that nearly killed me. One of the resulting symptoms was necrotizing fasciitis, most commonly referred to as the "muscle-eating bacteria." According to my doctors, in a culture plate of regular bacterium, it would take about three days to grow a quarter of an inch. Meanwhile, the clostridium septicum culture in my body took fifteen minutes to grow a quarter of an inch. My dad then explained the analogy that the doctors had relayed to him: it was the equivalent of someone standing on train tracks with a piece of paper to shield themselves from an oncoming train.

Because there was so much uncertainty surrounding my situation, this gave way to rampant speculation and rumors. Did I take steroids? Is that how I contracted the bacteria? Or was it a spider bite? Was I contagious? The media began to form their own baseless conclusions. Journalists took liberties with my delicate story, and they made assumptions that were wholly false and unfounded. Foran High School students who I had never met were being quoted as if they were my personal biographers. They did not know me, and I did not know them. Instead of following up with my surgeons, my parents, or with me, some writers created stories with the sole intent of garnering readers, even if the stories were not true. As I dwelled on questions that had no answers, I was angered at the media's lack of respect for my situation. I was still a human being.

The media coverage notwithstanding, the outpouring of support I received was incalculable. Whether I was sleeping or awake, there was a constant line to see me. One visit, in particular, reaches out through my memories. She was my friend's mother.

"How are you doing," she asked, trembling as a tear began to stream down her face.

Tears soon welled up in my eyes too. With a smile on my face, I held them back and told her, "Do not cry for me; I will be just fine."

Endless corrosive thoughts threatened to eat away at my strong will. I was wearing a mask of personal strength. To outsiders, I was the jovial, inspirational John who had persevered through illness on the strength and support of his friends. To myself and my immediate family, however, I could be the introspective, emotional John who only allowed himself to look back on what had happened when he was alone. While I did not want others to think that I had changed, at times I was plagued by self-pity, staring off into the blinking, operating, hospital-room night and wondering why.

However, I could not bring myself to say those two words aloud. If I allowed others to see weakness, if I gave in to those self-deprecating thoughts that crept into my mind, if I embraced my situation as my being any different than I was before, then others would view me that way. My physical attributes had changed, but I was still the same friend, the same brother, the same son, and the same Foran High senior. Biology was still my favorite subject, and I still possessed a zest for physically challenging my body. Before I showed them what had changed, they needed to see what had not.

My family, meanwhile, dealt with the pain quite differently from one another. My mother and my sister were the managers, the directors of the traffic, the delegates who wanted to diagnose the problem so they could chart out their next move. They were like me. We all had really strong poker faces for each other and for the many others who cared about me. That did not mean that we weren't affected by it, devastated by it, hurt by it, but we kept up the façade of our family's strength.

Conversely, my father needed to keep himself occupied when he was not in my room. To pass the time, he would do volunteer work at the hospital, answering phones and making sure that people who were coming into the hospital were seeing the appropriate doctors. The pain of coming so close to losing his only son, of being forced to watch him suffer through a tragic illness, and of knowing that his son's life would forever be affected by the events of one day took a far more noticeable toll on him than anyone else. What happened to me was the center of his universe, and it really controlled his mindset.

There were times when the tears were unavoidable, when I would break down, but as my prognosis improved so too did my attitude toward my predicament. What had happened to me was unfortunate, but it was not a death sentence. My condition was improving, and my doctors were encouraging me through my recovery.

"That's a pretty big bicep, huh?" I playfully remarked to Dr. Crum, the one who had removed my left bicep. He was examining the cavernous hole in my arm to ensure that it was healing properly.

He let out a guarded chuckle. "Yeah, Frank Zane," he said, referring to the famous body builder from the 1970s. I was just trying to make conversation, fishing for a funny response, searching for any form of normalcy in my unbelievable situation.

Thankfully, my left arm was spared from the same fate as my legs. But as much as I wanted to forget what had happened to me, my body had a cruel way of reminding me all over again.

"They're cold," I told my mother and my sister. I knew that my legs were amputated up to my hips; where they used to be only bandages now remained. These phantom pains came in flashes, flushing my body with the feeling of having legs and feet again.

Within two weeks, I had been removed from the ICU and relocated to the surgical floor. I was rapidly recovering, much quicker than any of my doctors initially had anticipated.

While my physical activities were limited, I began to work with a physical therapist to strengthen my atrophied muscles. Even though I had tried to test myself physically whenever I could, I had spent almost an entire month lying on my back. We started off with the lightest possible weights, between one and two pounds. Initially, I was insulted. Then, the realization finally set in; I was weak, a position I had never wanted to be in. My pride would have to understand that I physically was not the same seventeen-year-old who had lifted weights religiously throughout high school.

Sitting up and balancing myself became the focus of physical therapy. It was the only chance I had of being mobile. At first, I was like a baby just beginning to gain some independence. Wiggling my body up from the bed with my physical therapist's help, I would wobble to find my center of gravity until *plop!* And I would fall back down like Humpty-Dumpty. Eventually, I was able to steady myself for about thirty seconds; however, I was still unable to sit up under my own power.

How the hell am I ever going to live independently if I can't even get out of bed? I was frustrated, but it was more than that; not being able to do such simple tasks was degrading. After living my whole life unhampered by any physical restriction, I now had to relearn the most trivial details of existence. And that was only to sit up.

Even though my progress was not quick enough for me, I was close to being moved to a rehabilitation center—the last obstacle that remained before I could go home. I had to realize that I was not going to

17

wake up the next day and go back to school as if nothing had happened. My recovery was a long-term commitment.

While defeated thoughts sometimes challenged my will, I would not stop fighting, for the alternative was far more depressing—a life that was reliant on others to live it.

****

"Now I have to go see patients that are actually sick," Dr. Crum said following a routine checkup.

My smile was as wide as the sky. Less than three weeks earlier, when the last of the bacterium was scraped from my skin, the doctors were not sure if I would make it through the night. Now, with a clownish grin affixed to my face, I knew that I was getting better, that I was returning to normal.

With all of the limits that my predicament had placed on me, it would have been easy to give up. But I still had my goals that roused me each morning, the greatest of which was to walk with my class at graduation and accept my high school diploma. It might have seemed impossible, and maybe it was, but I believed in it.

After I got through everything at the hospital, I knew that I could start to learn how to do the things everyone else did—except, this time, it would be without legs. Sure, it would be a lot of hard work and how I went about it would be different, but it would be fulfilling for me to achieve the same outcome and live my new "normal" life.

So instead of conceding, I set a goal. I told my family that I wanted to walk with my class and receive my diploma. It was something I needed to do for them, for my friends, and for myself, regardless of how impossible it seemed. Even though expectations had been set by medical professionals—what I wanted could not be achieved—I gave myself a chance when few did. I saw value in my action. There was so much meaning in my pursuit of walking. Hope was my driving force because without it I had nothing.

In a life that was so different now and at a time when I was more self-conscious than I had ever been, I could walk up and receive my diploma like everyone else. I would not be left behind because I had changed. I would not be left behind because I earned it just like they did. I would graduate.

4

When I exited the elevator, my nostrils were immediately filled with that undeniable, undesirable smell, the one that requires a second flush and a spray after it. The hallways suffocated me with the asphyxiating scent of human feces. *Great, just what I need.* This, my home for the foreseeable future, was the floor that specialized in spinal cord injuries. It was Monday, September 20, 2004, my first day at Gaylord Rehabilitation Facility in the south central Connecticut town of Wallingford.

My day started at 7:00 a.m., when the nurse would administer my medicine before the doctors checked my wounds. Oddly enough, most of the staff did not want to touch my left bicep; so the responsibility fell on me to change the dressing before therapy. Even after a month in the hospital, my arm still looked like a shark had taken a bite out of it. At first, I had to bring myself to look at the gruesome sight. Regardless of its aesthetics, I recognized how lucky I was to even have my arm.

By about 8:30 a.m., I would meet my occupational therapist for a session that usually lasted between thirty minutes and an hour. We started our morning routine with me getting dressed. She would put a shirt, underwear, and shorts on my bed and turn her head. Lying on my back, I would lift my butt up in the air, slip my underwear on, and finally wiggle myself into my shorts. This was pretty easy, or it was until I tried to squeeze my body into the shirt. No matter how many ways I turned or how many angles I twisted, the shirt refused to go on. When I sat up and began to put it on, I felt like I was in a straightjacket. With my head stuck inside and my arms flailing, I lost the balance I never really had and fell over. Eventually, as I became more familiar with this new body of mine, I would be able to control it. However, those first few failures left me red in the face with embarrassed anger.

When I arrived at Gaylord, I was relying on a bedpan to go to the bathroom. Since I did not have legs to brace against the floor nor hamstrings to rest on the seat, going to the bathroom on a toilet was literally a pain in the ass. Although my occupational therapist intended to end my reliance on a bedpan, finding a comfortable position was almost as impossible as balancing long enough not to go to the bathroom all over myself. It was an acute pain that jabbed at my backside bones, like the feeling of sitting on cold marble for too long. I tried not to get down on myself; physically, I was not ready to reclaim my independence. I couldn't even wipe my own ass yet.

As if not being able to put a shirt on or use a toilet was not bad enough, my ring and pinky fingers on my right hand were debilitated. The contracture, or tightening of the tissue underneath the skin in my palm, was causing my fingers to curl inward. My occupational therapist and I both knew that if we were not proactive, the contracture could become permanent. To ease some of the tension in my fingers, she would warm up my hand with a heated towel or a paraffin wax before she would crank my slouching fingers to attention. While the solution seemed rudimentary, I trusted the professionals who surrounded me to remedy the issue.

Whereas occupational therapy worked to allow me to regain my ability to function on a day-to-day basis, physical therapy aimed to give me the strength to do so. In our early sessions, my physical therapist would tell me to lie down on an aerobics mat and then get back up. *Seems pretty simple.* No matter how much I rocked to try and gain momentum, I could not do it without her help. My atrophied, pastry-tube muscles had failed me.

How humbling it was to not be able to sit up on my own. No matter how well I might have been doing in my rehabilitation, in my head, my head that was moving faster than my recovering body, I was a laggard. Sitting up was a matter of strength, and the fact that I could not do it meant that I was weak. I didn't like the thought of me being weak, ever.

After a short break for lunch, there was a group therapy session. Held two to three times per week, they were typically light weight lifting sessions that lasted for about an hour. In the beginning, they were a necessary step in my recovery.

In my afternoon helping of OT, we continued working on my assimilation back into the real world. At first, I practiced in one of the many mock settings at the facility—a kitchen. Using a claw-like device, I reached for items that were out of my grasp; yet, I never liked using it. This kind of assistance made me feel incapable, but what other choice did I have? I could not climb out of my wheelchair and onto a counter every time I wanted something from the cabinet. Although I longed for my old life, I had to understand that certain aspects of it were going to be different.

Returning to physical therapy for one last reminder of how weak I had become, I continued to work on sitting up, except now my wheelchair was incorporated into the routine. From my chair, I would transfer onto the mat to practice sitting up and balancing my body. When I finally was able to push myself off of the mat after a couple days, I felt like I had completed the New York City Marathon. Then, I fell back to the mat and realized that my balance needed some more work.

On account of my tireless schedule, by the time I turned around, it would already be dinnertime. I would have dinner with whoever was visiting that day, and hopefully by about 10:00 p.m. I would be trying to get some sleep.

All of the therapy that I did in that first week was beginning to yield results. I no longer needed to brace my arms against the seat cushion of my wheelchair in order to balance. From abdominal exercises to rickshaw machine presses, my strength was steadily increasing. More importantly, this foreign body of mine was beginning to feel less and less unfamiliar with each passing day.

On Sunday, September 26, 2004, hundreds of motorcycle riders visited me at Gaylord. A friend's father had coordinated this charity ride to offset some of my exorbitant medical expenses. Starting at my hometown's Milford Showcase Cinemas, the ride was about twenty minutes along the highway. It would culminate with the riders pulling into the rehabilitation facility to wish me well in my recovery.

"Do you want a blanket or something to cover yourself?" my sister Jennifer asked. She assumed that I would be self-conscious, and in some instances I was.

As we headed toward the front entrance of the building, I looked at her, smiled, and said, "I have nothing to hide."

There I sat on the front steps of Gaylord waiting to greet these bikers. Surrounded by my family, close friends, and fellow patients, I would never forget the steady revving and rumbling of the motors on that fall afternoon. Watching the bikes ripple by like rising heat, I waited for the last biker in the endless line to drive through. Each engine had a distinct, discernible sound to it, a sound that I could feel through my body.

This would be my first experience with a crowd of bikers. All I knew of them were stereotypes that they were a lawless, rowdy bunch who lived and died by their own rules. Approximately three hundred bikers had made their way up the Merritt Parkway undisturbed and uninterrupted, an open-road drive facilitated by the police motorcade that had surrounded them. I did not know what was more ironic, the fact that these people who I had considered to be modern-day outlaws were cooperating with the police or just that these gruff-looking men and women were riding for me.

When I finally met the people who had ridden for me, they were not the stereotypical bikers I had imagined. Sure, some of them were dressed the tough part, but they were all down-to-earth, regular people, complete strangers who had taken time out of their lives to come tell me to "keep fighting" and that "we are pulling for you." One after the other, I shook their hands, smiled, and thanked them for their help and support.

A fellow patient who was sitting out there with me was a motorcycle enthusiast. He had suffered brain damage, but he was elated at the sights of the shimmering bikes that glistened in his eyes.

"His smile's the best we've seen it in a while," commented one of his family's friends.

While I was grateful for the outpouring of biker love that I received, I took solace in knowing that his day was a little brighter than before.

****

It took me about a week and a half just to be able to consistently sit up without any assistance. To hone my balance, my physical therapist and I would toss around a lightweight medicine ball. Regardless of if I was in my wheelchair or on the mat, she would hurl it at me and I would have to catch it and stay upright. This sliver of success, my first physical accomplishment beyond surviving, only emboldened my desire to physically push myself, so much so that I began using a universal exercise machine to work out my whole body. Gradually, and with great effort, my strength began to return and my technique improved.

My progress in physical therapy enabled me to perform more situational activities in occupational therapy. By my second week at Gaylord, I was grabbing plates from shelves, carrying pots and pans to the stove, and setting tables in the mock kitchen. There was even a living room where I transferred onto and off of sofas. While I knew I was not prepared to return home full time, the thought of attending my girlfriend's birthday in a couple weeks did not seem all that farfetched.

****

Although I was finally seeing tangible progress in rehab, it took my father longer to heal than anyone else. Mentally, I was leaps ahead of him; I would have to remind him that I was fine, that I had survived, and that what I was doing now was the easy part. My mother and my sister were able to see me doing more and more; they could see the improvement that I could see, that I could feel. It seemed like my father could not feel that way because he was doing the hurting for me.

Always trying to keep himself busy throughout my recovery, he made me a board to help stretch my fingers out on. It was the shape of turkeys that little kids make around Thanksgiving time by tracing their hands on construction paper. When he brought it into the room, I smiled and thanked him for the thoughtful and necessary gift. I would strap my hand onto this board and press down my hand to stretch my fingers whenever I was lying around in my bed.

****

In an effort to boost the morale of the patients, the facility would bring in social workers and psychologists to conduct group therapy sessions. I had never taken advantage of this program until Gus, a heavyset, Latino, double amputee in his early thirties, stopped by my room to pitch me on the merits of the meeting. This group, in particular, he said, offered amputees at the facility the opportunity to discuss their situations and to comment on their progress. Reluctantly, I agreed to go.

With melancholic and indignant tones, one by one the participants bitterly recounted their personal tragedies. They had not moved past their situations and were instead ruminating in their own misery. There was not an optimistic word uttered in that therapy session. *This is not helping my recovery; this is torture.*

My father turned to me with a surprised look. "Half of the people in here have lost a limb to diabetes," he said, "and the only food and drink they have to offer is coffee and munchkins! I don't get it."

These people were the stereotypes for people with disabilities; they viewed themselves as so different from the able-bodied that they inadvertently ostracized themselves from everyone else. I was not interested in looking back. I could not change what happened to me and neither could these people.

"Let's get the hell out of here," I whispered to my father. It was never lost on me that many of these people did not have the same support system that I did, but at the end of the day, self-pity was more superfluous than advice at the session. And I knew there was not a cure-all remedy for recovering from a traumatic experience. What worked for me might not have worked for someone else. I did not know how I would have reacted if I was middle-aged or even elderly; but I was still only seventeen years old with my entire life ahead of me. I also knew that healing came from within in accepting what had happened in order to move on. Some of the people in that room were not ready to take that step. That was the first and only time I attended a group therapy session.

****

At Norwalk Hospital for a consultation with the infectious disease specialists, I also met with my guardian angel Dr. Crum. While he was pleased with my recovery and happy to see me in good spirits, when I showed him my hand, his eyes grew critical and his brow calculating.

"If you keep doing what you're doing with your fingers, they're going to become clubbed. You don't want that to happen," he said, shaking his head. Behind my disbelieving eyes, I understood him. Clubbed meant curled, immovable, and permanent.

Faced with the possibility of losing further mobility, I wanted to tear out of that room like a tornado on a path of destruction straight for Gaylord. Why had my occupational therapist been so passive in her treatment of my fingers? Why had she not been honest about their current condition? *How could she do this?*

On Crum's recommendation my parents and I visited his trusted colleague, a hand surgeon that he worked closely with and that I had seen during my stay at the hospital. We told him what we were told: my occupational therapist at Gaylord had predicted my contracture would be resolved in a few weeks. In reality, he informed us, the issue needed two months of therapy at a much more intensive rate than what I had been doing. Two weeks had already been wasted, and my fingers had gotten worse. He advised us to have his occupational therapist make a customized finger splint to stretch my fingers.

As soon as I returned to rehab, my mother was fighting with my occupational therapist over the hand surgeon's conclusions along with my parents' decision to follow his advice. My therapist said that Gaylord could make a splint for me, but, according to her, the splint recommended by the hand surgeon was more than I could handle. Her disregard for the hand surgeon's advice was off-putting, but it was the reason why I was seeking an alternate treatment. The decision was made that the hand surgeon's occupational therapist would come to the facility early the following week. I could only hope that my doctors at Norwalk and my occupational therapist at Gaylord could come to some consensus on what was the best treatment for me. This was not the time for disagreement.

****

Like a little kid's ticket to Disney World, I received a day pass to return home for my girlfriend's birthday. Even if it was just for a day, it would take me away from the hospital setting. I wouldn't have nurses and doctors checking in on me; instead, I could socialize with friends and family in a house, not a patient's room. I was out, in the real world.

While I had done a pretty good job convincing myself that I would be able to transition from rehabilitation to home life, I still had my misgivings. How would others look at me now? Would people act differently around me? Could everything really be as it was before I left?

However, being in a family atmosphere quickly quelled my fears. Celebrating my girlfriend's birthday reaffirmed the principle that had taken me through rehab. I had not changed and neither had the way that people viewed me.

****

Outside of physical therapy, I started lifting weights to better prepare myself to live independently. While the side work was increasing my overall ability to function, it was also serving to motivate others around me. My father relayed the words of one patient who was paralyzed from the waist down to me.

"When your son is out there," he said, "I just want to work harder."

****

I had lost all faith in my occupational therapist at Gaylord. In trying to fix my fingers, she had led me astray, and now my contracture was as tight as a stripped screw. To remedy this issue, my hand specialist recommended the occupational therapist cast me for a new finger splint.

29

Tedious as it was, he instructed me to wear it for ten minutes every hour throughout the day. For full use of my fingers, however, it was a necessary nuisance.

While there was finally a concrete plan in place to deal with the contracture, I still could not comfortably sit down; whether I was in a chair or on the toilet, the pain was practically unbearable. Sitting in my wheelchair for extended periods of time was problematic as well. Even with the cushioned seat, I would eventually begin to slouch and then have to reposition myself on the chair. I knew that my body would have to get used to my new seating situation, but there had to be a way to alleviate some of the pressure on my bottom bones.

Conveniently, I was scheduled to see a prosthetist within the facility during the week. He was going to make me a seating bucket, or a socket, to relieve the stress I was putting on my back as well as my bottom. To do this, he cast the remains of my lower body. The expectation was that the socket that this prosthetist created would serve as a precursor to a more comprehensive prosthetic device. However, when I asked about the possibilities, he was noncommittal. Even with the uncertainty, I remained optimistic that I would be able to walk by the time graduation came.

From the moment we were finished, I was anxious to see what he would make for me. Days later, when he presented it to me, my anticipation quickly turned to angst. The socket came out like a plastic corset that went up to my stomach just below my chest. The bottom was not even rounded to capture the shape of my great butt; instead, it was just a flat base.

Where am I going to put myself in this thing? Hoping that my initial judgment was rashly conceived, I hopped in. The socket was more uncomfortable when I was in it than when I wasn't. *There has to be something else, someone else who can make this work.*

There were not many prosthetists who had worked with a patient like me, maybe not any. Sensing the angst that adorned my face, my parents were reassuring throughout the process, constantly reminding me, "We will get you whatever you need." They were going to find someone who could develop the device that was right for me. I knew they would.

5

Anxious thoughts had been running through my mind since we left Wallingford and headed southwest to Milford. This was the first time I would be seeing my community in an ordinary, public setting. And I was embarrassed, not because of my predicament, or because of the news presence, or because I was out in a social setting with my peers. No, I was embarrassed because I had a big, beat-up, pink clunker of a wheelchair that was loaned to me. It was not the manly entrance I wanted to have at my Foran homecoming.

I just wanted to watch the game like any other Foran High student on the field that night. In my current predicament, however, this was not possible; so, Foran made me a special entrance and allowed me to watch the game with the players on the sidelines.

As I wheeled myself out to the field, my face was brighter than my fluorescent wheelchair. I couldn't help blushing. I felt like all eyes were on me. I would have rather done a naked lap around the track than be watched by everyone. Holding back my emotions, I cheered on my buddies, and for a moment, I was like every other kid around me. In the middle of that endlessly opaque October night, Foran sent the crowd home happy with a win.

I ended up staying home in Milford the entire weekend. Being in my room returned me to a state of normalcy. And my own bed never felt so good.

Before, when I had visited my girlfriend for her birthday, I could not even get into my own house. The front porch was in no way handicapped accessible; now, I could come in through the front door. However, without the help of an old, childhood friend, it never would have been possible. His mother and her boyfriend had reached out to a local Home Depot to see if they could offer me any assistance. As it turned out, the local Home Depot had heard about my story and was more than willing to help. With a ramp in place, I no longer needed to be lifted up and down steps. I was not a burden anymore. I was home.

****

It had been months since I had taken a shower, not the Wet Wipe rubdowns I had grown accustomed to, but a real shower. There was only so much of my musk that those moist towelettes could cover up.

When I had virtually forgotten what a shower felt like, a waterproof stretcher was prepared for me to use. As the water spurted from the showerhead and cascaded over my body, I lost myself. I was a kid playing in the summer sprinkler. I was a traveler weathering the spring showers. Embracing the warm beads that dripped from my face, for the first time in two months I felt clean.

****

Nearing the conclusion of my stint at Gaylord, I was guardedly optimistic that in another week I would be able to move back home. Before that could happen, however, I needed Dr. Crum to approve my release. Based on my progress, I assumed that this was merely a formality.

The contracture on my ring finger had improved since our last visit and was beginning to loosen up. My pinky, meanwhile, I had conceded as imperfect; regardless of the therapy, it was going to lose some range of motion. However, I could not see this as a viable reason to keep me in rehabilitation.

Pointing at the portion of my left bicep that met the elbow joint, Dr. Crum said, "What the hell is the matter with your arm? There's a big hole there!" His tone was dry and he was trying to be humorous, but there was nothing funny about this latest setback.

My mother had incessantly asked my doctor at Gaylord why my arm was not healing properly. It looked like a hard, scabbed-over golf ball, but he would say that it looked "fine." Now, Crum explained that the initial skin graft had failed to catch over my elbow joint and that it would have to be corrected before he could authorize my release.

His words were a verbal fasciatomy, cutting into my confidence and leaving me vulnerable. I would have to go back to Gaylord. Between the doctor who did not recognize what a healing skin graft looked like and the occupational therapist who did not know how to loosen the contracture in my hand, I felt let down. They had let me down. *One minute I think I'm going home. Now, I'm going back in for surgery.*

Crum scheduled me for a skin graft the next day. Just as the doctors had done the first time, a layer of skin was taken from my stomach and placed over my inner elbow. Due to the precarious position of the graft, my arm was immobilized on a board to prevent it from bending. The six hundred or so stitches in my arm were counting on it.

****

"I cannot officially recommend someone to you," a representative from the Amputation Coalition of America (ACA) said to my mother, "but, off the record, if I had to see someone, it would be Erik Schaeffer."

From the very beginning of my ordeal, my parents had promised to get me the best care that was available. As we pulled out of Gaylord on our way to Hicksville, NY, we hoped that this prosthetist could offer me an opportunity we were not even sure existed.

When I wheeled into A Step Ahead Prosthetics, I did not feel like I was in a stuffy doctor's office. The waiting room was open and inviting, and the secretary was personable. Prosthetic limbs rested on pedestals, pictures covered the walls, and framed newspaper clippings told the stories of patients' triumphs. *Will I be up there one day?* Those pictures that formed an inadvertent collage on the wall were truly inspiring. Jovial, young children being able to walk for the first time, adults of all ages and predicaments given a new lease on life, and athletes competing at the highest level, all because of this prosthetist.

Naturally, my father initiated conversations with patients in the waiting room. He took great pride in the fact that his son had survived this traumatic experience, and he needed to preach it to anyone who would listen. It was like he was stuck on repeat. Sometimes I just wanted to shake him until he stopped.

"Enough with the story already!" I yelled to him. I lived it, I knew it, and I didn't want to hear it again.

From the moment we met Erik, we were struck by his poise. We discussed the use of "shorties," which were short prosthetic limbs used to ease the transition to walking with longer limbs. These prosthetic devices were supposed to make it easier to balance and get the hang of the motions of walking.

"Forget that." There was no indecisiveness in his voice, no question about what was best practice for dealing with an amputation level as severe as mine. "We don't use them here." Then, he showed us what A Step Ahead Prosthetics did use.

Opening a swinging door, Erik led us into the island of misfit prosthetics. Hundreds of prosthetic casts surrounded us, while outlines and sketches of devices lined the workbenches and tables. This was his workshop where he weaved dreams into realities and allowed his patients to realize feats that they never thought were possible. *This is our guy.*

Already sold on Erik's abilities, he took us on an elevator to the second floor. *Now, he's showing off.* Walking through the "skin tone room," we saw where artists worked to create synthetic skin to transform prosthetic devices into seemingly real limbs. From hair to veins to nails to creases and wrinkles, these artificial skins were flawless. They covered legs, hands, ankles, wrists, and even fingers. For me, the synthetic skin was not as practical, nor did I really care about having legs that looked real. For others, it eased the self-conscious concerns that might arise when wearing a prosthetic in public.

We had brought my first socket, the plastic baby swing, along with us. Erik literally took it, threw it up on his desk in an embellished and sarcastic manner, and mocked it.

"Listen, this a joke," he said, in a very matter-of-fact tone. There was not a doubt in his mind that he could make something that was "one thousand times better" on his first try. His demeanor quickly changed from joking to serious before we had finished laughing. "Are you up for the challenge?"

After I said yes, he looked at me with the conviction of someone who was confident in his craft.

"You're gonna fuckin' walk," he said. Going from a guy who was ill prepared to deal with my needs to someone so self-assured in what he could provide for me, my family and I knew that Erik could help me. The image he exuded was reassuring yet realistic. I believed in him.

I told people from the beginning of my stay in the hospital that I wanted to go to rehabilitation so I could get home. Remember that I went from "able-bodied" to "disabled" in one night, so, in my head, I had something to prove. Just because others didn't expect something of me didn't mean I expected less from myself. I really felt like if I didn't push myself and take ownership of getting myself strong again, no one else would.

That is not to say that every waking moment at rehabilitation was successful. The biggest disappointment I can remember was not being able to sit up. I would go back to my room and be so upset with myself and with my lack of progress. Sitting up was a simple task for everyone besides me, and I was reminded of how far I had fallen. I was not the spry, athletic kid I had once been, and it would be a while before I was again. For me, this moment was a wake-up call that my recovery was going to be trying. Humbled by my inability to get myself off of that bed, every day I came back and tried harder. Instead of letting it drag me down, I used my "failures" as motivations.

While I was accountable for my recovery, walking was something that I couldn't do alone. So when rehabilitation ended and I met Erik for the first time, it was like a shot of adrenaline. His confidence in what he could provide for me made me feel like I had no excuse for not meeting my goal. This was just another instance where an aspect of my life aligned to reinforce and support my goal of walking with my class at graduation.

In any trying situation, the easy part is acknowledging that a tough journey is ahead. What is difficult and what I have realized is that truly successful people can look at obstacles and see opportunities. In the beginning of rehabilitation, I could have given up on myself because I was not strong enough to sit up; yet, I knew I needed to do it to regain my independence. That was the ultimate goal, the one that all of the others reinforced.

Erik, meanwhile, could have said what other prosthetists had said before—"You will never walk again"—but he saw this as a way to greatly impact my life while also challenging his skill. What it comes down to is that there is no comparison to the feeling of overcoming a challenge and proving to yourself what you are capable of.

6

Three months had passed since I was first hospitalized, but those three months could have been three years. Among the excruciating surgeries, the uncertainty of knowing if I was going to live or die, the agonizingly slow pace of rehabilitation, and the emotional toll of the whole process, I was still the same John. Now, I needed to apply the skills that I had learned at Gaylord in the real world. There were only so many mock cars to get into, so many jars to reach for, and so many stairs to scale. On October 30, 2004, I signed myself out of rehab.

As we pulled up to the house, something felt different. It had been so long since I had lived there. Even with my periodic visits back to Milford while I was in rehab, now it was real, it was permanent.

My dogs, a burly German shepherd and a pudgy Boston terrier, fumbled over each other to sniff my forgotten scent. I wheeled my way over to my room. The bed was all I cared about as I dismounted from my chair and lay down. Rolling around in my bed—not a hospital bed, not someone else's bed, my own bed—I realized the feeling I had longed for. I was finally home.

****

Since I was forced to take control of my rehabilitation early on in the process, I thought that nothing got done right unless I did it myself. This mindset allowed me to work my way out of Gaylord and maintain my independence along the way. Admittedly, I had a chip on my shoulder the size of my old body—a five-feet-six, healthy, seventeen-year-old kid. But that's all I wanted to be again—a kid.

Being home did not preclude my rehabilitation from continuing. Instead, I had an outpatient physical therapist come to my house to work with me. Before she could assess my progress, she needed a baseline to determine what our focus should be. So we went into my kitchen and she handed me a broom. With both of my hands, I held it horizontally in front of me as she pushed downward on it to gauge how much I could resist her. She even made me curl various cans of food. *Cans? Brooms? How are these exercises relevant to my recovery?*

At Gaylord, I felt restrained by the pace they had me work at, but this level of in-home therapy made them look like the hare. And I would always be the tortoise if I kept working with physical therapists who did not push me. I needed someone who was going to work with me, someone who was going to challenge me, and, most of all, someone who could keep up with me.

Like a bad date doomed from the first greeting, the in-home physical therapist knew that our time together would be brief. After that first session, she recommended Jim Ronai, a local physical therapist, to me. His office was conveniently located right around the block from my house.

****

When I first wheeled into Rehabilitation Associates, I had my doubts. *What groundbreaking perspective could they possibly offer me that the other physical therapists could not?* I expected the worst because, up until that point, no physical therapist had challenged me enough to prepare me to reach my ultimate goal of walking again.

As I sat in the waiting room with my eyebrows furrowed and a scowl on my face, I thought that this guy would be like all the rest. Many therapists had never seen someone, at any age, in my predicament. Then, I met Jim. He had this calm, reassuring demeanor about him. "Don't worry," he told me, "we'll make it work."

40

While I did not even have a seating prosthetic yet and I was unsure if a walking prosthetic for my amputation level existed, the prospect of walking to accept my high school diploma motivated me.

"If you want to walk," Jim said, "then we have some work to do." While I was still uneasy, I could tell that he was different than the others. He had a plan.

After a ten-minute warm-up on an upper body ergometer, which was essentially a stationary bike for my arms, we took steps to strengthen my abdominal and back muscles. With me lying on the mat, Jim would hurl a medicine ball at me. Like a pendulum, I would crunch up, catch the ball, extend my arms behind my head, and throw it back to him.

Similar to my time at Gaylord, my sessions with Jim also included the parallel bars. While I could move along the bars with the ease of an Olympian, he wanted me to extend myself beyond what I had already done. I saw this when Jim asked me to perform dips. With no legs, I had the advantage of weighing less. However, after a set, he began to incrementally add weight to a belt attached to my waist. As the pull on my waist grew heavier with each upward thrust and my arms began to burn, I was roused by Jim's challenge. He was demanding the most of me, pushing me as hard as I pushed myself.

The work that we were doing together made me feel closer to my former able-bodied self. Both inside and outside of therapy, I was beginning to get back into my old routine. At home, my weight lifting regimen brought me back to before my illness. I was charting my own progress and putting in extra work because I knew it would help me reach my goals. Before I could walk, though, I first needed the means to sit down.

Returning to A Step Ahead Prosthetics, I was scheduled to be cast for a seating prosthetic. It was a unique dilemma because, in most situations, a cast was made by wrapping the limb in plaster. For me, however, Erik recognized that he had to shape the socket precisely to my dimensions; so, he designed a platform with sliding boards on it that pressed me from different angles at the same time. He needed to see how I responded to the varying arrangements so he could find which angles relieved the most pressure. It was a tiring process, but Erik promised me that, within a week, I would have a seating socket ready to wear.

He was a man of his word. When I visited him the following week, he had produced a socket that was incomparable to the Jack-in-the-Box one I was in before. The sleek, slender, shiny plastic lining conformed to my body, curving up my hips and around my waist where two laces waited to be tied. After I tied myself in like a shoe, I pulled the socket's second layer—a carbon fiber shell—over the interior liner and ratcheted down the ski straps that were affixed to it. Tighter and tighter the socket squeezed me to compensate for the surface area I lost from not having any residual limbs. One last click…and then, for the first time since my amputation, I sat comfortably.

I could have cried, but I could barely breathe. The socket had to be fastened to my waist excruciatingly tight so that I did not move in it. This left the skin around my hips chafed and sore like hands on a chin-up bar. Tolerance was the price of comfort.

Now that Erik had the socket designed, he had to figure out how to adapt it to support prosthetic limbs. While it was a work in progress, it was still progress.

I never felt so happy to see my home than that first time I came back from rehabilitation for a weekend visit. It had been so long since I was able to relax in a familiar and comfortable place. Having a taste of normalcy made me appreciate what had been provided for me by my parents all along.

42

I always wanted to be treated the same as I was before, but it was hard to do so living in a hospital and rehabilitation facility for months. As much as I tried to act like the old me, I was still confined to those buildings and to the routines that came along with being there. Once I was finally back at home, I felt a weight being lifted off of my shoulders. To take what I had learned in rehab and adapt it to the real world meant that all of the hard work I was doing was worth it. I saw myself becoming more independent at a time when it mattered the most.

Outpatient physical therapy began with the purpose of preparing me to walk, but the first time I met Jim, I didn't want to give him a chance. Coming out of rehabilitation where I set a more aggressive pace for my therapy than my therapist did made me feel like I was better off on my own. While I thought Erik could do something for me that I couldn't do myself, I was skeptical about what Jim could offer. I was wrong.

Not only did he understand how to help and challenge me, but he also helped me to expect more of myself. At this point, my mindset shifted. I never thought about my limitations anymore; instead, I realized that I could do just about everything I wanted to, albeit a bit differently. Ultimately, the end result was still the same.

Since the early stages of my illness, I had embraced and quickly adapted to these changes in my life. I learned that the small choices I made on a daily basis turned into habits, and eventually, those habits affected my character and outlook. If I solely focused my thoughts on having to go about living my life differently and did not see the value in what I was doing, I would never be happy. And happiness is a choice.

7

From the beginning of my stay at Gaylord, my father had looked forward to my homecoming party. He would constantly remind visitors, friends, families, and even strangers that when I was back home, we were celebrating. I think that it allowed him to see the light at the end of the tunnel for me. Even if he had, at times, moved slower than me in my recovery, the thought of me being home again comforted him.

While I never wanted to be the center of attention, I came around on the party when I realized how important it was for everyone to see me in my recovery. Most of my visitors in the early stages of my hospitalization thought they would never see me alive again. Now, I had made it home to my family and my friends.

When the day finally arrived, the weather was dreary, with an overcast sky, a penetrating cold, and a hard ground. However, no forecast could have kept the herds away. Outside, under the heated tents in our backyard, my family hosted approximately 250 people. The constant flow of people shaking my hand and wishing me well reminded me of my stays at the Norwalk and Gaylord. These were the same people who were by my side from the beginning. Their unwavering support had pushed me to work harder every day; I had a responsibility to them, just as much as to myself.

****

Jim was showing me that progress could be made, not just on my own, but with the help of others as well. He had surrounded me with an unbelievable crew of therapists and aides. I could feel their genuine concern for my well-being. The upbeat atmosphere at Rehabilitation

Associates dissolved my misgivings about physical therapy and, with it, my abrasively self-righteous attitude.

However, therapy was not cheap, and after three weeks of working with Jim, my family's insurance provider no longer wanted to cover my daily visits to his office. In an act of incomparable generosity, the owner of Rehabilitation Associates permitted me to rehabilitate myself until Jim felt that I no longer needed it. This man showed unbelievable compassion in allowing me to make appointments for physical therapy, most of the time free of charge. Without the constant and consistent help of people like Jim and his boss, my transition back to everyday life would have been that much more difficult.

****

My return to everyday life was not limited to just the physical aspect of it. To ensure that I graduated on time, I was homeschooled in English, calculus, anatomy, and physics. Between three and five times per week, I was taught each subject for an hour or so. It was by no means as mentally taxing as the regular classroom, but it was what I had to do in order to get back to the high school hallways. After all, it was my senior year.

****

My parents had been with me through my toughest moments and had dealt with the realistic possibility that I would die on multiple occasions. They were instrumental in my recovery, having come with me to every doctor's appointment, every physical therapy session, and every occupational therapy session; anywhere I was, they were not far behind. They had been my advocates when the doctors said that I would never walk again; they had been my protectors when my contracture was not healing; and they had been my parents when I opened my eyes and realized that my life would never be the same again.

Now, I needed to function on my own; however, my parents were understandably reluctant to let me go. While they always wanted to help, their help would only end up holding me back. I did not want to be dependent on anyone else. The only way for me to learn how to live was through failures and successes. *So don't hold that door open for me, don't reach up to grab something from the top shelf for me, don't help me up the ramp, even if I look like I can't get up, don't help me up.* I would adapt and live independently.

8

Sitting in the car with my parents, my heart raced along the highway. *Can't we go any faster?* It was the night before Christmas Eve, and I was giddier than a child restlessly anticipating the morning. I was getting the new pair of legs I had asked for.

****

In that eternal second, no breath was exhaled, no movement was made, not even an eye blinked. *Those are my new legs!* While words were slow to trickle from my mouth, I looked the legs over from toe to waist. From the metallic ankles to the storm-gray shins up to the blue-rubber knees into the raven femurs, joints then connected the legs to the socket itself. Like a person at about three feet tall, this futuristic device stood next to me, and I waited for it to start walking on its own. The prosthetic even had bendable knees that would afford me the ability to sit down when I wanted to. Through the joints to the knees down to the mannequin feet, these were the closest a person could get to real legs without actually having legs. And they were mine.

Once the interior socket found its groove in the exterior casing, I clamped myself in with the ski straps. *And there they are.* Dangling below me were my legs. I had legs! Still in awe, I thought about this extra weight where my actual legs used to be and how unnatural it felt. They were not physically a part of me, but at the same time they were.

"It's going to take some time for your body to get used to them," Erik warned. He was cautioning me about the wear the walking prosthetics would inflict on my hips. Eventually, my skin would develop calluses, but "you're just going to have to work through it and gut it out for a while," he said.

Then, I remembered that I actually had to put my body in there and stand up. It would be the first time in four months that I would be standing upright, and my emotions were muddled between nervous and excited. *Can I even do this?*

Erik helped me into my wheelchair, and we made our way into the open-floored waiting room. Here, a set of parallel bars sat in the corner waiting for me to test my new legs on. *Will these things really be able to support my weight? Am I too top-heavy?* For as many fears as I had about lifting myself up and falling flat on my face, I had to do it. This was the moment that they had said would never happen.

Grabbing on to the bars above me, I pulled myself up. *I'm standing.* I did not have to imagine the legs in front of me swinging one after the other. They were there. This was no longer a simulated "walk along." I was walking all by myself, letting the natural rhythm of my step propel me. Left arm forward, right leg kick. Right arm forward, left leg kick. I repeated this motion, applying what I had learned in exhaustive hours of physical therapy for that one moment, a time forever ingrained in my memory.

Before my parents, before Erik, before his secretary, I was doing the impossible. As I moved along those parallel bars, Erik saw his hard work realized. While I did not know that I was doing it, he was impressed that I was already performing an advanced gait movement. Naturally, when walking, the leg extends forward, the knee bends, the foot hits the floor, and then the process starts all over again. While a below-the-knee-amputee was expected to exhibit this kind of gait movement, I was not. Instead, my walk was supposed to resemble a more rigid, polio-like manner. And that would have been fine by me because I still would have been walking.

Feeling my way along the bars, I moved toward my waiting wheelchair and eased myself into it. The parallel bars gave me a sense of security. They were safe, immovable, cemented into the ground. However, on graduation day I would not be walking with them. I knew that if I intended to accomplish my ultimate goal, I needed to use forearm crutches.

With my father and Erik each holding an arm, I was up on my feet again. Then, Erik was running off. Before I blinked, he was back with a set of crutches and I was letting go of my father. Like a spectator from atop a building, the ground seemed so far away. As I looked down, I was standing on my own, three feet higher than I was used to, with only two foreign pieces of metal keeping me from crashing back down to earth. *Holy shit! I'm going to fall!*

My heart was a bass drum first beating, then booming, until finally blasting, throughout my body. There I stood uneasily on my technologically advanced stilts, wobbling and trying to balance myself. I was afraid to fall; I was afraid to even take a step. *It's just like walking in the parallel bars. Push down with one arm and use your opposite hip to swing the leg.* But it wasn't. I could trust the parallel bars. With the crutches, I had to believe that the prosthetic limbs would support me. And I did not. Like a deer in the headlights, I stood, helpless and unable to move.

Looking me down from head to prosthetic toe, Erik said, "Try and balance yourself without the crutches now."

As I handed off the crutches to my father, I felt like a flag blowing in the wind. I was all alone up there on my legs, powerless against my own body. Bobbing back and forth just long enough for Erik to snap a picture, I shakily tried to maintain my balance before I was helped down. This would definitely take some getting used to, but at least I had hope. Mere months after I was told it was not even a possibility, walking was now an attainable goal.

****

Hanging around A Step Ahead more, I learned about amputees and the varying levels of amputation. It quickly became clear how having residual limbs affects one's functionality. Most people have a tough time differentiating between an amputee who does not have legs and someone who only has a part of his/her legs, or residual limbs. I did not have any residual limbs. I did not have a knee, a thigh, or any part of my femur; there was nothing but my hips. And my hips and my butt were supposed to be the muscles that propelled my prosthetic legs into motion.

A below-the-knee amputee uses the typical walking gait because of the mechanics of his/her knee. The knee provides a natural rhythm to walking from the bending, the flexing, and the extending of the muscles to controlling how the foot hits the ground. Above-the-knee amputees have residual limbs, their thighbones, to use with a prosthetic device. The natural extension of the thigh provides substance to allow the technology of a prosthetic knee to be used. Even the unilateral hip disarticulates that Erik had worked with in the past had the comfort of their own limb on one side. It was theirs. They could trust it to brace them against the ground. Meanwhile, I had to put all of my trust in these artificial limbs that were standing in, in place of my lost legs.

****

Christmas might have come early for me, but my family's tradition still remained the same. Every Christmas Eve, my great aunt hosted the annual family get-together. Always a memorable occasion, this year's party was particularly special to me.

Up until that day, I had exclusively worn gym shorts. Now, looking down and seeing denim molded around my legs, even if they were not real legs, made me feel comfortable. It made me feel normal.

What Erik had been able to do for me was a miracle. Yet on that Christmas Eve night, he had allowed me to do something far more meaningful than anything I had done up until that point: I was able to stand up and take a picture with my entire family. Of all the dreaded family pictures, where complaints extended beyond the flash of the camera, that was the most compliant, even eager, one of all.

****

Jim planned to hold a 5K charity run on Sunday, April 3, 2005, to commemorate my hard work and dedication to my recovery. While I did not need a pat on the back, I was honored and planned to walk a lap around the track. Although ecstatic, not surprised, over my determination, he knew, just as I did, that we had work to do if I was going to have a shot at fulfilling such a lofty goal.

****

After the holidays, the gloss of having the legs wore off; now, I had to learn how to use them. While Erik had told me to strap them on as tight as possible, I was still experimenting with how tight the interior socket had to be. Once it was laced up, there was the process of securing the carbon fiber exterior over the plastic socket. If it was not aligned properly, my weight would be unevenly distributed and I would feel added pressure on my hipbones. This inequity could also affect my gait. Even if I was able to satisfy all of the prerequisites for securing the prosthetics to my body, I still had to deal with the friction they created on my hips. Whether they were too tight, too loose, or just right, the prosthetics left me with road rash-like scrapes. It was as if I was sliding on gravel in a Speedo.

Besides the physical damage the prosthetics were inflicting on my hips, my hands were as raw as tenderized meat from the generic crutches that I was using. After gripping the cylindrical handles for a few minutes, my hands would quiver with pain.

While the sores would eventually heal and the ache would ultimately dissipate, I was suddenly unsure of myself. Was walking really going to be such heartache and struggle? Was it worth it, if every step that I took hurt me?

The very moment that I saw my prosthetic legs, I was awestruck. All of the work that I had done with Jim and on my own was for this. My parents' eyes filled with pride further reaffirmed my belief in myself.

My emotions were endless—accomplishment, relief, motivation, joy, even fear. After being told I would never walk again, I was putting on legs and standing taller than I was before. I saw myself taking steps in between the parallel bars feeling that familiar sense, that motion I had never forgotten. It was like riding a bicycle.

At the same time, I was worried about disappointing all the people who had rallied behind me. I had done this for them just as much as for myself. While I had walked with the assistance of the parallel bars, I couldn't bear the thought of not being able to take a step on my own that day. I had to remind myself that my journey would not be highlighted by instant gratification. Walking, like sitting up, would have to be relearned.

With the legs, a new and exciting element was brought to my sessions with Jim. I remember being anxious to see how everything would go now that I had them. Early on, my eagerness got the best of me. I had zero experience with prosthetics and was completely ignorant to how challenging and physically taxing it would be to operate in them. Yet my expectations were as if I was still an able-bodied, physically fit teenager. Walking was walking, right? I was unprepared for the frustration of what I perceived as minimal progress. Worse, the pain I experienced just squeezing myself into the socket and taking a few steps was comparable to circus performers walking on glass.

Although I was comfortable in the parallel bars, I did not have this security with the forearm crutches. As much as I tried to maintain my belief in myself, I began to doubt my ambitions. The thoughts of professionals who had said that walking was an impossibility returned to me. Sometimes, I thought they were right. I imagined them saying, "You won't be able to do this," "This is a lost cause," or "You should've given up on this idea months ago." Since Erik had built the legs, I hadn't learned or done anything new to change the outcome. I considered giving up and residing in a wheelchair for the rest of my life.

In this time, I was my own worst enemy, driving myself with expectations and feeling disappointed when I did not meet them. It was one of the hardest things, but looking at the situation from afar, I realized that each step was a small victory. It reminded me why I was doing this in the first place—to walk at graduation with my friends, to be like everyone else there that day. This understanding played a major role in overcoming my doubts. In the same way, it is the small tastes of success that will help you overcome self-doubt and stick with what you need to do in order to reach your goals.

9

It had been nearly eight months since I had attended a class at Foran High School. My memories of before I made it back were of an uncertain life, of learning how to sit up, of getting the privilege to visit home for a day. While I had spent restless nights suffering through a very adult situation, I wanted to crack jokes with my friends in the cafeteria, move through the hallway in motion with everyone else, even interact with a teacher in a classroom setting. I wanted to be a seventeen-year-old kid again, and once I had finished my home-school instruction I could be. When classes restarted the first week in January, I would be restarting with them.

****

Going through my usual morning routine of brushing my teeth, shaving, showering, getting dressed, and doing my hair, I felt like myself. However, there were naturally going to be some differences outside of the obvious physical ones.

Because the pain of being in my prosthetics was still too fresh, I would not be wearing them in school. Foran was receptive to my needs, as Principal Cummings made any and all concessions to assist me in my transition back.

Since it took me an inordinate amount of time to do general, functional activities like taking a shower and getting dressed, I was permitted to come in late in the morning. Meanwhile, my schedule was abbreviated to include only the major academic subjects required to graduate. This meant no extra electives that could hamper my reintegration back into school. It was quite the contrast to my senior classmates, many of whom had conveniently loaded their final quarter of high school with inconsequential classes.

Unfortunately, in my situation, I was deprived of the greatest privilege of senior year: being able to drive to school. While I had options, they certainly were not the *coolest* of choices—one being that I could take the bus. That would have been too much of a production because they would have had to send one of the small, accessible buses with a wheelchair lift. I was trying to fit back in, not completely stand out.

My only real option appeared to be the usual ride from one of my parents. They had been ferrying me around from appointment to appointment for months, and I appreciated it every time, but this was different. This was high school. Even in my predicament, I did not want to be the senior who was dropped off by his parents. Nobody wants to be that kid, the one who gets kissed on the cheek by mommy and then has to retrieve his lunch in front of all of his friends after he forgets it in the car. It's embarrassing!

When I arrived at Foran, I did not expect a hero's welcome, and, to my delight, I did not receive one. The last thing I wanted was for my school community to feel sorry for me. While my classmates and the school were sensitive to my situation, they did not view me as a story, they did not make me feel unwanted, and, most importantly, they did not make me feel different. I was no different than any of them; only the situation I had to deal with was. As people and friends passed by like subway cars, I was still just another face in the crowd. The train flow of the hallway had not passed me by though. Instead, I felt like I got on right where I had left off.

That first day might have been the only time in my life that I was actually excited about calculus. In that third quarter of school, I was one of the few seniors who did not already have raging "senioritis." Most of the kids could not even be bothered with their mandatory academic classes, let alone their electives. My situation was a bit different. I had been away from the classroom for months, and I savored the return to the familiar format. I could have been stuck in an advanced-level college course on the most beautiful summer day, and I would have been content. Homeschooling simply was not the same.

I had never considered handicap accessibility as a fully healthy teenager. I did not expect my classmates to clear the halls when I came by. It was not like "Watch out, the guy in the wheelchair's coming through." However, if there was a crowd congregating in the hall and making traffic, my friends and I would playfully yell, "BEEEEEP!" until the congestion dissolved. We were obnoxious like that at times, but we were seniors and we could get away with it. Overall, my interactions with friends and others at school did not revolve around what had happened to me. It just was not a topic of conversation. I never said a word about it; I did not discuss it, and I did not let it affect me in front of them. Personally, I would sometimes have my intimate struggles within, but my demeanor and my upbeat attitude reminded Foran that, despite what had happened to me, I was still the same person.

While I was settling into the life of a teenager, I maintained contact with Erik and continued to meet Jim for PT sessions at his office. Crutches were the topic of conversation. In those first few weeks with the prosthetics, it seemed as if every generic model that I tried put more strain on my hands than the last one. Inflamed and irritated, my fingers looked like Vienna sausages and my palms were as red as clay. The only way that I was ever going to be able to walk was through practice; my body would never take to the prosthetics if I was not working in it. After letdown upon letdown, I wondered if there was a crutch out there that would ease some of the excruciating tension in my hands.

The crutches were integral to my mobility. Without them, I could not walk, so my mother went on a mission to find a pair that worked for me. As luck would have it, she discovered a set of crutches with ergonomic grips. They were different than the previous pair, which had standard cylindrical handgrips. This change in design would enable me to distribute the weight on my hands more evenly. From the first day that I tried them, I knew that they were the right pair for me. They allowed my hands to withstand the weight and pressure that I was exerting on them. However, I soon recognized that just because I had found crutches that would provide my hands with more comfort did not mean that walking would be a Sunday stroll.

I continued to work tirelessly with both Erik and Jim to learn how to position my weight in the walking prosthetics. While I had little difficulty using the parallel bars to walk, the difference between the bars and the crutches was like having legs and not having legs. Within the parallel bars, I could lift myself up from the seated position and not have to worry where they were going. When I attempted to replicate the reciprocal gait movement I had done my first time in the walking prosthetics, it felt natural.

With the crutches, however, this was not the case. Not only did I have to watch how I held them, but I had to pay attention to where I held them as well. There was practically a checklist to follow just to take one step. As I was ambling up, I asked myself, *What's in front of me? Where are my feet going to land?* One crutch then the other went, as I alternated the step of my crutch to the swing of my hip.

My hips felt like they were up against a cheese grater with each step. The friction was excruciating at times, and because of it, I could only tolerate the walking prosthetics for roughly fifteen minutes at a time. This plodding progress I was seeing was beginning to wear my patience down.

Naively, I had expected a quicker adjustment even though the strides I was making were unheard of.

Coming home one day after physical therapy with Jim, I talked to my mother and my sister about my doubts. "Maybe the doctors were right [about not being able to walk]," I uttered in a defeated, unfamiliar tone. I felt like such a failure; I was letting everyone down.

However, neither was disappointed in me. "No matter what decision you make, you need to do what is best for you," my mother and sister said. Instead, they were supportive as they had always been.

"If walking is too much right now," my sister Jen began, "then don't do it." A simple choice? No, but I had pursued the unbelievable to realize it, not to wither under it.

As the days passed, my tolerance for the prosthetics grew, and I knew that I had to continue on. I began to walk around my house after physical therapy sessions. From my kitchen to my living room, I went back and forth. The pain was becoming more manageable now; my desire to walk, to complete the lap in the 5K and to accept my diploma, drove me to take each step and tolerate the hurt.

While the walking prosthetics were physically becoming easier to wield, I also had to prepare myself mentally. These "smart legs" had the ability to sense when I shifted my weight backward. If I leaned back too far, they would bend so I could sit down. To ease my mind when I was walking, Jim would attach a small strap to my waist to catch me if I fell. Yet this did little to mediate my misgivings. Whether I had a leash on or not or if I was inside or outside of the facility, I did not feel confident in my ability to walk with the crutches. Familiar feelings of uneasiness that had paralyzed me on Christmas returned to me. What if the ground wasn't flat or if I crutched into a pothole? I was afraid of falling, but really I was afraid of failing. *Who will pick me up if I can't pick myself up?*

The answer had to be that I would rise, and I would rise again and again after that, as many times as it took. My disability would not define me. I would walk.

10

Swimming was meant for staying cool in the summer, certainly more of a leisure activity than an exercise. Or so I thought.

That first day at the pool, my lungs burned with the noxious, thick chlorine vapors that hung in the air. I wheeled over to the swim team's bench and transferred off of my chair. Hopping down onto the tile, I used my arms like crutches and swung over to the water's edge. When I threw myself into the water, the cold penetrated me to my soul and I felt that instant jolt of being in the water for the first time. Then I was sinking, lower and lower like a penny in a pond.

****

Upon Jim's recommendation and in an effort to further my endurance, during my second week back at Foran I reached out to an old friend and one of the best swimmers on the team, Chris Mahoney. While there was no practical swimming prosthetics for my amputation level, he was receptive to the idea of training me.

"[Swimming's] usually done by someone who isn't facing your physical challenges," Chris said. "But it doesn't mean that someone with your physical challenges can't do it."

****

Even before my amputation, I was just an average swimmer. Now, in my present condition, I had to learn how to swim all over again. I had plenty to learn from Chris.

Trying to keep my head above water and feel out this new aquatic world, I did my own version of the doggy paddle.

Once I was able to steady myself, we began to develop my stroke. We started out with the basic freestyle stroke. For me, there was nothing basic about it. After three or four strokes, I needed to somehow breathe without gulping down water or losing my balance. Each time I tried, however, my head bobbed up and my butt sank down.

"Get that butt out of the water," Chris chided me like a seasoned coach. He wanted my body to resemble a "U," explaining how this curved form would help me control my body when I needed air in the water.

I felt like a piece of driftwood aimlessly floating through the water. Finally, after completing a lap, I stopped at the end of the lane to take a breather. My arms, which were as heavy as cinderblocks, needed it. In the placid pool, enveloped by the warm, encompassing air, I could have even dosed off.

Chris's voice, however, sounded the alarm, waking me from my conscious slumber. "Turn around and keep swimming!"

When I pulled myself up on the ledge and out of the water that first day, I could not imagine myself swimming more than three hundred yards. Muscles I had never felt were shaking under the shiver of a cold fatigue. As tired as I was, I knew the feeling would eventually subside as I became more comfortable with the exercise. And with that, my endurance and agility would increase as well.

While Chris did not have experience working with amputees, he approached our training as he would with any other novice in the pool. "This is more about you gaining confidence," he said. To him, it would broaden my view of exercise. "Swimming is your first cardio activity, and it'll allow you to see beyond the weights."

Day by day, we worked on my stroke and how to breathe in between it. To the swimmer, it was all about efficiency. Naturally, Chris wanted me to make sure I was "pulling in" as much water as possible. Each stroke became the longest, length-of-the-lane stretch I could muster; with my hands cupped, I tried to capture as much of the pool as I could.

From twisting my body in the opposite direction as my stroke to keeping my butt in the air to maintain buoyancy, I learned there was a science to swimming. The process was as mechanical as a metronome with multiple moving parts clicking to the rhythm of my hands clapping against the water.

"You should feel like you're gliding through the water," Chris said. While I was not yet as graceful as a swan, soon enough I would learn to glide.

****

There was never a second thought or consideration about attending college. It was a forgone conclusion. My ambition was not derailed by the events of the past six months. Instead, my goals were galvanized by my desire to not let my predicament limit me. I had always planned on applying to local schools, such as Southern Connecticut State University and the University of Connecticut. Now, it became that much more important because of what had happened to me. I needed to find a place that was far enough away so I could still move out but close enough so I could return home if I needed to for any reason. That narrowed my list of schools down considerably. Nearby Fairfield University in Fairfield, CT, emerged as a potential option.

****

Shifting my weight from one side to the other, I practiced swinging one hip into the step while keeping the other hip in place. It was such an unnatural feeling at first since I was only using my hips to produce steps, and I could not feel my feet because they weren't actually *my* feet.

I constantly had to remain conscious of how far I leaned back. The idea of my legs giving way without warning left me on alert. Struggling under the adversity of my misgivings, I did not want to be perceived as weak. However, Jim saw beyond my machismo to recognize

66

my hardship. With him standing behind me waiting to catch me, he and I practiced how far I could lean back without toppling over. Still, my uneasiness lingered like the ache on my scarred hips.

The question became could I actually complete the quarter mile at Jim's 5K benefit run. It was a valid one; I had never walked anything close to that amount, as I still did not have the stamina to intensively train in my prosthetics. I still feared stumbling and, in this case, becoming a speed bump during the race.

Although my doubts degraded my confidence, conceding to the challenge was not a consideration. It couldn't be. I had made a promise to Jim, and whether I successfully completed the lap or I failed trying, I would be there on Sunday.

11

The air's breath was damp and the ashen sky was unsure of what it wanted to do that day. Later, I was expected to walk a lap around the Foran High track. Although I was anxious to put the techniques I had practiced in physical therapy into action, my emotions were clouded with a mixture of apprehension and anticipation.

The modest success I had seen in my toils and triumphs, through my breakdowns and breakthroughs, palled in comparison to the lap. This actually mattered. There would be no parallel bars, no strap attached to my waist, and no Jim waiting to catch me if I fell. I had to prove that I was capable of doing what no one thought I could do.

****

By the time the entrants started to register for the race, the sun had cleared the clouds and enlivened the sky with its rays. Bustling with participants, volunteers, and supporters, the cafeteria was swarming like the beach on the first day of summer.

"Time to start the show," Jim said. When I heard those words, the thoughts of all the *coulds* dissipated from my head.

****

Stabilizing myself against the crutches and with the race gun in my hand, I stood behind the runners. Jim held the megaphone to my mouth.

"On your mark!" I shouted. "Get set...Go!" The shot sliced through the air and runners ran into the morning. Now, it was my turn.

****

When Jim and I made it down to the track, music blared in the background and a crowd of supporters swelled. Yet in that moment, there was only the track and me. No distractions or doubts could break my concentration as I stood up from the golf cart and gingerly began to move my legs. One foot after the other I kicked, conscious of each step that I took and cognizant of the way the crutch touched the ground. Because of my plodding pace, I could feel the mass of people build up behind me like someone staring at you when you sleep. Nobody wanted to pass me. They must have thought it would be a crime against humanity.

"Don't worry," I called back to them playfully, "it's going to take me A LOT longer, so go on ahead." With a laugh, the crowd started to make its way around the track.

Trying to stay focused and conserve my energy by allowing the prosthetics to take some of the burden off of my hands and arms, with each step I gained more confidence. A quarter of the way around the track, I boasted to my father who was walking next to me, "I'm going to be able to finish this. Maybe I'll try and do a second lap." However, my mind was moving faster than my body, and this proved to be wishful thinking.

As I trudged toward the finish line with sweat dripping down my face, my body felt like I had just walked fourteen miles. Months of tiresome rehabilitation, of self-questioning, of anticipation for that day tumbled down my face.

I called out into the crowd of friends, acquaintances, community members, and people I did not know, "I would not be where I am today," the megaphone echoed, "without the help and support of every person here. Thank you for everything you've done for me."

In just four months of work with my walking prosthetics, I had defied the initial (and minimal) expectations of experts in both the medical and prosthetics fields and completed the lap in about fifty minutes. The time was not important, though. What I had done was. Walking was no longer an uncertainty.

****

The atmosphere in Rehabilitation Associates the day after the race was triumphant. What I had done we had done together.

"Great turnout, great atmosphere, and you were awesome! I'm definitely going to do the 5K again," Jim said. There was a pause that sat in between us, the void occupied by something unspoken waiting to be said. "So I was thinking about it," he hesitated, "you want to walk the entire two miles next year?"

To him, there were no questions or limits to my ability. I was not an anomaly to him; I was not some medical miracle who was defying the odds with each step. I was just a regular guy working his way back from a trying ordeal.

"You think I can do it?" I stammered with uncertainty rattling through every word.

A smirk streaked across his face. "There is no question in my mind that you can," his calm, yet stern voice said. His words shot through my chest like adrenaline, piercing my heart and changing my worldview. Jim had always believed in me; he had more confidence in me than I did in myself. From that moment, I could finally see that there were no "cans" or "ifs." These words were simply unnecessary impediments in my quest to live a healthy, active, and normal lifestyle. I was going to be able to do this. I *would* do this.

12

With an amputation level as severe as mine, there were more uncertainties about my independence than actual truths. Confidence was the one constant among all of the unknowns. Yet my confidence was not enough if I wanted to walk more than a lap. I needed another physical therapist like Jim, someone who was equally as sure of himself as he was in his ability to work with me.

"I have the perfect guy for you," Erik said. "He's a crazy old bastard, but he can help you."

This physical therapist and trainer was Dave Balsley, a fearless professional who pushed himself just as hard as those he trained. At nearly sixty years old, he had recently competed in arguably the most grueling ultramarathon there was. The three-day Badwater Footrace spanned 135 miles from Death Valley, Nevada, to Mount Whitney, California, with temperatures that reached as high as 130 °F. After learning this not only did I respect him, but I thought he was a crazy old bastard too.

Based near Central Park in New York City, Dave would have me over to his apartment once a week. While I would continue to see Jim, Erik wanted to bring in someone who he was familiar with. Dave, with his extensive experience in training amputees, would collaborate with Erik to grow my functionality in the prosthetics. Charting my progress, he would make recommendations to Erik about techniques I was learning and adjustments he felt needed to be made to the prosthetics.

****

Thoughts of falling unavoidably penetrated my mind. I had always either pulled myself up on the parallel bars or pushed myself off of a stationary wheelchair. Now, Dave wanted me to stand up from a bed using only my crutches. It wasn't the physical pain I feared, though. It was the failure.

"Your dad and I are standing right here in front of you, John," he encouraged me in his slight Southern twang. "Let's go! You can get up."

As I started to rise, I fell, and as I rose again, again I fell. Eventually, I stopped the dance and was able to bring myself to standing. But there was no time to rest on my crutches.

"What're you doing just standing there?" His twang had become taught, almost disappearing, and his tone was serious. The idea was to go right into walking.

I wasn't about to argue with him. After all, this is what I wanted. Stiffly, I moved one crutch forward as if it was stuck in the mud. Then, my hip kicked and the opposite leg lurched in the same direction. Thrust. Lunge. Thrust. Lunge. My eyes never left the ground. I had to be sure nothing was in front of me. Really, I had to make sure that the prosthetics would hold me up. This drew my upper body forward and left me resembling a powered-down robot. In my stubborn refusal to defer to the prosthetics, my shoulders sank and my back strained under the stress I was putting on my arms. I had to learn that I could rely on these legs that were not mine.

"Tartaglio, you ever try to swing through with your crutches? I talked to Erik, and he thought it was something helpful too," Dave said. My puzzled facial expression replied that I had no idea what he was talking about.

The motion was like someone using crutches with an injured leg, he explained. Unlike the reciprocal gait where I walked with one leg at a time, I would now use both legs. And I would go faster. In theory, there did not seem to be much of a downside; yet, as we discussed this new technique further, I started to realize that I was about to set out on the most grueling walk of my life.

With Dave's encouragement, I planted my crutches into the ground, kicked my legs out in front of me, and went…NOWHERE. *What a letdown. All of that for a distance I could spit farther than.* My next attempt had to be better. It just had to be. Throwing my body into it, I curled my abdomen and lifted my feet through the air.

TWACK! Just as quickly, my feet smacked the floor. I had practically stayed in the same place.

Bracing myself against the crutches, I felt weak. "John," Dave said, "hold yourself up and try and balance." The fear that filled me was the same fear as when I stood without crutches for the first time in Erik's office the night before Christmas Eve. *Can I do this?*

With my arms erect, my feet no longer touched the ground. And then I was falling, slowly, gracefully, violently like a skydiver without a parachute. In Dave's arms for that moment, my heart was pounding so hard it might have bruised my chest. I was shaken up, but I wasn't beaten.

Mustering up the courage to hoist myself up again, I lasted a few more seconds before I fell back into his arms again. And when I tried again, my step grew to a half of a foot! Although it wasn't the long jump, I felt accomplished. Eventually, with practice my gait lengthened, but still there was a hesitance I struggled to overcome—a fear of what could happen.

****

Steppers? My face scrunched up like a wrinkled shirt. *The ones mothers use?* They acted like stairs, Jim explained, allowing me to learn control, balance, and how to approach steps when I encountered them in the real world. It sounded promising, but my confidence was deflating quicker than a tire on a winter day.

Reaching deep down inside for some guts, I pushed off the crutches, thrust my abs forward, and prayed that I landed on my feet. When I opened my eyes, I did not have a concussion, and I was not in a hospital bed. Standing atop the stepper looking over Jim's head, I realized I had done it! I wanted to throw my arms into the air in celebration, but I recognized that I would have fallen if I did.

Then, reality returned, and it was not giving me a pat on the back. Jim wanted me to hurdle over the stepper. Unlike before, I did not feel the pangs of an impending catastrophe. If there was ever a time, it was now that I needed to follow through on this leap of faith.

Vaulting forward, my stomach turned as I launched myself into the air, unsure of where I would come down, how I would come down, or if I would come down. Before any other thought could register, my feet hit the ground and I stood tall on the other side of the stepper.

As those two feet touched the ground, there were so many questions I had answered within myself. Up until that point, I had been hesitant to put my trust in my prosthetics. That day, however, I had confronted my fear of falling, my fear of weakness, my fear of failure, and I had persevered. I finally believed in those legs that were not mine.

****

The sounding bell signaled the end of the day as the hallways flooded with students from all directions. My mind was on the Bridgeport Bluefish game later that night. The independent Atlantic League team had offered me the chance to throw out the first pitch, and the last thing I wanted was to airmail the ball over the catcher's head or, even more embarrassing, to throw a weak two hopper to the plate.

To my complete surprise, a news team from Michigan that supposedly was following me around school for a local report actually worked for Oprah Winfrey's Harpo Productions. I was lucky enough to have the support of so many members of my community, but this was ridiculous; now, even Oprah was on my side.

****

I scrambled down to the away team's dugout while they warmed up and put on my legs. And with the signal, I was up and walking onto the field.

On the mound, I looked to home plate. With the incandescent lights overhead, the spring chill descended onto the field as the catcher took his position behind home plate. In his crouch, he smacked his mitt, opening and closing it. He was ready. I was ready. Cranking my arm back, I steadied myself against the crutch and followed through. In that silent second, the cameras flashed and reality was suspended in the moment the ball leaped from my hand. And there's the pitch...

Right down Broadway, the ball smacked against the leather, STRI-IKE! Standing there in the center of the diamond, the stands blinked like a strobe light and the ballpark shook with applause. As I waved to my supporters, I said a silent prayer to myself:

Thank you, God, for not letting me look like an idiot.

13

Hurdling down the hill behind the auditorium, the security guard whipped me around like a shopping cart. After the rollercoaster had stopped and I opened my eyes, I was in the middle of the football field, isolated and with all eyes on me. I had thought I would be going out with my classmates, like any other Foran student. Instead, there I sat, the center of attention that I never craved to be, but who over the past months I could not avoid being.

As I looked at the masses that filled the bleachers, these were all people who I had met at one time or another. Without their support in a time when I needed it the most, without Erik's prosthetic genius to do what had never been done before, and without Jim and Dave's relentless drive to bring out the best in me, a return to where I once was would have been that much more difficult. However, without my family it would have been impossible.

My mother's *work first, worry later* attitude gave me a model to help manage my physical and emotional adversity. She committed herself to my recovery and enabled me to pursue my dream of walking again in spite of what doctors and prosthetists told her. My father was my biggest fan, taking pride in my perseverance and never missing an opportunity to tell someone how proud he was. And Jen, my sister, allowed me to feel comfortable with who I was. She knew that I would be OK because underneath the bandages, the scars, and the sometimes-faux smiles was still her kid brother.

It was the early afternoon, when the sun's rays had relented and a cool breeze had descended over the football field, when the ceremony began. In the glistening navy sea of classmates that had begun to file out of the auditorium and fill the rows on the field, there were no social boundaries. Cliques had dissolved in the shared, uncertain feelings of what we were leaving behind. Some would venture to schools far removed from comfortable Connecticut. Others would stay local. Some would go straight into the workforce. Others would join the armed services. We were all going somewhere, just not together. This was the realization that high school was about to end.

The moment might have been melancholic. But as my best friend and Class President Mike Lynch addressed the "greatest class to walk through the halls of Foran High," his tone was promising. To him, the future was infinite with possibilities. New goals to be set. New experiences to be had. New relationships to be formed. And old ones to leave behind. Then, looking at me, he said, "Dealing with tragedy can make us better prepared to deal with challenges in our future." In the wake of my situation, we had all grown up.

The gears of graduation began to turn. One by one, students walked across the field to become graduates, and the ebb and flow of rows rising, names being called, and diplomas being accepted commenced. With a nod of the head from the teacher assigned to my row, everyone stood and lined up.

This was it, the time I had waited for, worked for, suffered for, and the day that I knew would come when I first woke up in the hospital. Mike asked me if I needed help getting up, but I shook him off. Setting the brake on my wheelchair, I gripped my crutches and hoisted myself into the air.

There was no turning back now. With my eyes fixated on the ground, I flailed my crutches forward and began to leap in the direction of the stage. The air erupted as if Foran had just scored a touchdown, and chills prickled up my spine. Even with my focus solely on retrieving my diploma, the crowd's support was a transfusion I felt flow through me. One last swing remained—only inches separated me from my goal—before I grasped the presenter's hand, accepted my diploma, and exhaled. Countless hours of surgery, days in limbo between life and death, innumerable minutes of physical therapy sessions, and monotonous months in rehabilitation were all for this moment. Fulfilling my promise ten months in the making, I had done it!

Behind me, as he had always been, was Mike, who raised his fist into the air in a solemn salute to me. Slaps on the shoulder and handshakes were unending as I sat and watched the rest of the ceremony in awe of the moment.

"Will all students please rise for the last time," the principal commanded us. There was finality in his voice, and the field went silent. "The Joseph A. Foran Class of 2005," he paused, "you are graduated!" Instantaneously, the ground shook with applause before a frenzy of flying caps flew through the air.

As the sun bled across the horizon, outstretched hands reached for the falling hats and day began to turn to night. Once the pictures were taken and the congratulations were exhausted, we left the field that day never to return as high school students again.

The magnitude of what I had done began to set in. When I was in the hospital, my greatest fear was not if I would survive, but if I would be physically capable of leading an independent life. I had done what neither doctors nor prosthetists believed that I could do; I had walked. And I would continue to walk because it was not an award that I wore around my neck. It was a practice of everyday life, the normal existence I strived to live.

It was such a great feeling to be with all of my friends at graduation and share the day with them like I was supposed to before my illness. To stand up, walk, and receive my diploma felt like such a breeze compared to the quarter mile walk I did at the 5K run that Jim held for me in April.

But it was not about the distance that day. That day allowed me to reflect on what I had set my sights on while I was lying in a hospital bed months earlier. It let me see that even when I was faced with adversity, an obstacle that was said to be impossible, I was able to succeed.

In walking at graduation, I started to understand how to accomplish what I wanted in life and what it would take for me to continue to be successful. When I was wracked with fear and doubt, I had to dig deep and remember why I valued this goal. Bringing normalcy to my life drove me to never give up.

14

The honking horn from the rusty, early nineties Jeep in the driveway told me that it was time to go. I lifted myself out of my wheelchair and into the passenger's seat and quickly disassembled the chair and my friends tossed the parts in the trunk. After a slap of the hand and a "What's up?" the Jeep was in reverse, rumbling out of the driveway on the way to one of that summer's many high school graduation parties.

"Dude, this may sound weird," he stammered, searching for the right words before he cleared his throat, "but I forget that you're even in the chair." I'm sure my friend did not realize how much this simple statement meant to me, but this was always how I wanted others to view me. While I was physically different, who I was had not changed.

My unflappable desire to be no different than the next person was reinforced by Jim, Erik, and Dave's equally assured belief that I could do as much as I wanted to do. In their own ways, they had each radically challenged my bleak prognosis to give me opportunities instead of outcomes.

****

"Have you ever given any thought to competing in a triathlon?" Jim asked. I did not even know what a triathlon was, but his inquisition enlivened my competitive sense and I wanted to know more.

He explained to me that a triathlon was an endurance competition that consisted of individual sports—swimming, biking, and running—combined into one event where the winner was determined by the fastest cumulative time. Since I was neither strong enough to leg out the run nor did I have any form of practice on a modified bike, Jim suggested that we do it as a team. He could do the bike portion, while I would swim, and Jackie, another physical therapist from his office, would run.

"Do you want to do this?" he asked me.

I was so eager that I practically fell out of my seat responding with a resounding "Yes!" When I thought about it, I was as excited as I was nervous. While I was confident in the work that I had done with Chris, I did not know how that would translate in the triathlon. How would I stack up against the other competitors? I did not want to let Jim and Jackie down.

In training, I kept my goals modest. While I did not expect to win my event, I did expect to compete. Being able to swim the half mile was not the accomplishment. Rather, taking pride in my effort and the result of my labors was. My stamina was quickly accumulating that summer. Before two weeks was out, I was swimming a thousand yards. Now, I just needed it to feel like fifty yards instead.

****

It was the third week in June, and I was on my way to A Step Ahead for a routine checkup. Sitting inside of the examination room, I could hear other amputees working outside the door and the chatter between those who had accompanied them. Most of Erik's patients were like me—ambitious, competitive, and goal-oriented. But unlike them, there were no certainties and no baselines because my situation represented the baseline.

Erik and I discussed what was next for me—triathlon, how I was preparing for it with Chris, and what my expectations were. He was a good listener, but he was a much better talker. Licking his lips and then cupping his hands, there was clearly something on his mind.

"Have you ever thought about running?" Erik said.

Up until that moment, running was not even a daydream in my mind. I had only seen running prosthetics a few times, but before our conversation I did not think they were an option for someone with no residual limbs. Had there ever been someone with my amputation level who had run? I shook my head at a loss for words, subconsciously anticipating what he was about to ask me.

"Let's just say that if I could make something, would you be willing to give it a shot?" Erik was offering me a new means of mobility in spite of all of those who had said it would never happen. There was not a doubt in my mind. Armed with his prosthetic know-how and my determination to live life without limitations, we would write our own history together. And we would succeed because we believed in each other.

From the way that he was talking about it, he seemed like he had already plotted out a plan to create this device. He had.

"Me and Dave have been discussing it and have some ideas," he said. With the socket already developed from my walking prosthetic, Erik had a place to start from. Collectively, they did not want to have two legs hitting the ground like the walking prosthetic and they did not want the legs to be free-moving. It needed to be as light as possible to lessen the burden on my body while also giving me the most speed. As he spoke, the great potential of things to come swirled around my head. I would be able to run! On the streets, on the track, in triathlons, maybe even in Jim's 5K next April. Before my mind could run rampant with possibilities I never knew existed, Erik brought me back from the clouds.

"I want you to become a member of Team A Step Ahead," he said in the same collected tone he had when he first told me that I was going to walk again. He was giving me a chance to be a part of a team again, to compete across the country in events that were not exclusively for people with disabilities. Athletes who had achieved remarkable accolades because of what Erik was able to do for them looked at me from the wall. They were now teammates of mine.

By the beginning of July, Erik had produced the running prosthetic that supposedly did not exist. With Dave's assistance, Erik came up with the idea to have two femur shafts branch out from the socket and connect to one central piece. This centered piece was the median between the prosthetic femurs and a handlebar that had two small, C-curved flex feet attached to it. They reasoned that having two feet instead of one would not only give me more stability but also more bounce from my spring-like feet. Unlike the walking prosthetic, I would not have to worry about landing evenly on two separate legs. My balance would also be assisted by the proximity of the running feet to one another. Together, they would offer me the support I needed to push off and shoot into my stride.

The only problem was that the running legs did not have knees. So when I was locked in, I would be unable sit down. While this could make it difficult to run alone, Erik was confident that this was the best design for me to start with. My attitude: You make it, I'll try it, and we'll figure it out from there.

Leaning against the examination table, I gripped my crutches and pushed onto my new legs. There I stood, straight as a string bean; at first, I wobbled trying to find my balance.

"Look, it's Tigger!" Erik yelled. Everyone shared a laugh, and after a few minutes of feeling the legs out, I began to move around. Not fast, but faster than I had. I was not the gimp Michael Johnson, but I was no longer a statue either. I could run.

If you were to tell me when I was fifteen years old that I would be doing endurance events, I would have laughed and called you crazy. To be honest, I hated doing cardio workouts of any kind since the mile run in gym class when I was young, and that carried on into my teens.

So what the heck made me start? It comes back to how my past experiences shaped what I value now. I achieved success in a way that professionals never thought would be possible by walking to receive my diploma; in the same sense, learning that I could compete changed what I valued. Without the idea to do a triathlon thrown into my head by Jim and without seeing the amazing people who Erik had helped accomplish remarkable athletic feats, I would have never tried an endurance event.

From having the right people around me to being on track to attend college and pursue a career, the aspects of my life were aligned to reinforce my goal of competing. It meant that I could live a life that was even closer to what I had before. This was more than normalcy, though; this was living life without limitations.

15

The sky was as clear as Caribbean water. Walking on the street alongside of me, Jim talked about how far I had come—from the guarded, stubborn teen who had pouted in his office to the confident, open-minded young adult who now stood next to him.

He asked me how excited I was for college and my first triathlon, the Madison Jaycees sprint, which was set for the first weekend in September. Bringing me on with him and Jackie for the competition was an easy decision, he said, because, "I'm like a rock in the water." After a laugh, he became quiet.

My shoulders were beginning to slouch. I wondered if this walk, which had turned into a trek, would ever end. Then, it did.

"John," Jim said with prideful exuberance, "you've graduated from rehab." His sobering words lingered like unwanted silence. We both knew this day would come; yet, even with the progress I had made, it never seemed imminent.

When I was first released from Gaylord, I had an attitude that said it's me against the world, and if you're not with my program, then get out of my way. After a few visits to Jim's office, however, my demeanor changed. Not only did Jim have a plan specifically for me, but he cared about me as well. He wanted me to achieve my dreams just as much as I did, and he pushed me to do more than I ever thought was possible for myself. I realized that if I wanted to make it back to where I had been, I needed to let others help me get there. With the dedicated support I received from Jim and his office, I no longer had to be an army of one.

Physical therapy was no longer a necessity. I recognized that and Jim did too. He, along with Dave and Erik, had put me in a position to live a life as normal as any other person. I could stand, I could walk, I almost could run, and I could live independently. I would be on my way to college soon enough.

As the days passed by and turned into weeks, I thought about the 5K benefit Jim and I were holding the following April. After the inaugural race concluded, Jim had asked me if I was up to the task of walking the two miles around the track the next year. He did not doubt that I had the dedication to prepare myself physically and mentally for the test. And neither did I after I accepted the challenge. However, my situation had changed, and I began to wonder about the possibility of running the entire 5K.

****

Just yesterday, it seemed, I was walking to accept my high school diploma. Now, the truck was being loaded with duffel bags of clothes, toiletries, snacks, lamps, pillows, and generic blue bedding. My mother, my father, and I were squeezed in there like a clown car. It was a short drive over to Fairfield, but my parents were already missing me even though I was still in the truck.

We arrived to the commotion of parents honking their horns and kids standing off to the side, embarrassed by the mere presence of their guardians. It was move-in day. I saw kids who looked like me carrying nightstands and laundry baskets into and out of dorms. Like ants working to complete a task, families hurried through held-open doors and into tunnel corridors. Momentarily, they would disappear before they reemerged empty-handed and sifting through the rest of their belongings.

Assembling my wheelchair, I grabbed the handle by the door and swung myself into the chair. I felt like any other kid there, lost in the confusion of leaving home behind, taking boxes of my life and lugging them into a communal living area surrounded by complete strangers.

Walking down a dimly lit hallway, the new carpet smell had not yet aired out. There was an unspoken awkwardness that lingered in the hall, and it had nothing to do with my physical situation. Parents smiled as we walked by looking for my room. Shy students looked at the floor, some offered a "What's up," but there was that feeling of not knowing what to expect. Everyone was as green and new to this place as the next person.

As we walked up to the room, it was like a boom box blasting sound from the moment we walked in. "You ready for this, roomie?" Mike, my best friend and college roommate, had already arrived. Clearly, he was easily excitable.

After we were unloaded, it was time for our parents to go. With the good-byes starting, I noticed that my father was not in the room. Then, I heard him in the hallway.

By the time I came out of the room, it was as if the entire floor was his audience. Tomatoes sprouted from my cheeks. Proud as he was of how far I had come, it was embarrassing. I did not want to be the story all over again in college. All I wanted was to be like the next guy.

Everyone was looking for a friend those first few days of college, someone, anyone, who shared some common interest to relate to. Mike and I were lucky that we already knew each other, but there were plenty staring down at their plates in the cafeteria.

Although we began to build relationships with the guys on our floor, in the back of my mind, I could not dispel the thoughts that some of the people I was interacting with would be tempted to ask me about what had happened. In no way was I bashful about my experience, but I took exception with the way some people went about approaching the subject. If the first question someone asked me was "What happened to you?" I would generally respond with "Nothing, what happened to *you?*" To me, there was no difference between us. It was a bit dehumanizing when this happened because they were clearly judging me based on my physical predicament. I was not "disabled" in my eyes, and I did not want anyone else to treat me like a charity case.

However, it soon became evident that college girls do watch *Oprah*, and word travels faster than Amtrak when somebody is on her show.

During that first week of school, a girl who lived in our dorm ran into our room squeaking, "Hey! You're that kid that was on *Oprah*, right?"

I looked at her from my desk, almost in disbelief that she knew who I was, before I smiled.

"That's me," I said with a shrug.

This girl did not give any indication that she knew anymore about me than the next person, and I did not press the issue because I did not want the attention. Quickly, though, the news of what had happened to me circulated around the dorm. It was unavoidable; I could not hide behind all that I had been through nor did I intend to.

****

Wheeling in through the front doors of the "Rec Plex," or the student gym, I swiped my student ID and noticed that the floor was filled almost entirely with good-looking girls chugging away on elliptical machines, treadmills, and bikes. *Not a bad place.*

When I got off the elevator on the basement floor, I could hear the faint sound of classic rock playing against furiously blowing fans. My senses were heightened by the typical locker room stench that filled the hallway leading up to the weight room. I was ready to work. Then, it was like the record player abruptly came to a halt. Any excitement I had was diminished by the lack of a ramp to get into the weight room. It was only a few steps, and I could have hopped down, but it was the principle of the matter. I was alone, and I was not prepared to MacGyver down the stairs in my wheelchair. Luckily, I was able to get a lift from two guys, but not having a handicap-accessible ramp left a bad taste in my mouth.

This place is an armpit. As I looked around in disbelief, I was trapped in a time warp. The most modern piece of equipment among the relics was an abdominal wheel that was probably purchased in the early eighties. Rusted weights lined the mirrored walls that dripped with perspiration. There were lifting machines with snapped pulleys, battered weight benches, cracked weight plates, and busted barbell clips. At that moment I recognized that, if I intended on training, not just for the triathlon, but for the functional life I would continue to lead, I needed to find an accessible facility. Clearly, the Rec Plex was not highlighted on the tour for prospective students.

I did not live in social fear; if I did, this journey would have been much different. I knew that once people actually got to know me, they would drop labeling me as "disabled" and I would just be John. That's how it was in high school, at least.

Mike was a big part in helping me with that. We would hang out with and befriend the new acquaintances each one of us met at Fairfield. And when I met someone for the first time, with or without prosthetics on, I carried myself as if nothing out of the ordinary had happened to me. I was there to do the same thing as everyone else: work hard and play hard.

16

My wet suit hung from my closet door, reminding me of the competition that lay ahead. The distance, a half-mile swim, was not a concern; my training with Chris had prepared me for it. Still, I was nervous. The Madison Jaycees would be my first triathlon and, overall, my first competition since I was on the Foran football team.

Over the past year, I had been driven as much by my desire to return to my former life as I had been motivated by the expectations of the strangers and friends who were pulling for me to succeed. Now I owed it to Jim and Jackie to do my best and to prove to myself that I could still compete. Race day had arrived.

Slipping into my seal-colored suit, I packed my bag with towels and a few pairs of goggles, and I grabbed a bagel for the road. The early birds were not even awake, but the bleak, blue morning cold was. The race was scheduled to start at 7:00 a.m. at the Madison Town Beach in local Madison, CT. So off we went, into my mother's truck on our way to the race.

I did not expect to win my leg of the triathlon. However, I was not making the trip to come in last. I had worked to give myself the ability to compete with able-bodied and disabled athletes alike. Last was not an option. No matter how prepared I felt, I needed to prove to myself that I could do this.

****

The water was still and the sun skimmed across the surface like a skipping rock. It was almost time to begin. This was my moment. With roughly three hundred competitors encasing me, I tried to size myself up to them. Any prerace jitters had worked themselves out, and I was confident as I moved toward the shore.

Shaking out my arms, I felt the goose bumps rise up from my skin when I entered the water for a quick warm-up. It was always cold at first.

"Will all entrants please assemble at the starting line," the race coordinator announced. "We're about to get started."

With his word—"Go!"—athletes stormed the beach. As they were rushing ahead of me, I could not help but wonder how much easier this would be if I were running too. Instead I was using my arms like crutches, swinging my little butt forward until I hit the water.

My sole concern was my place in the race. Then again, that was the pressing thought on everyone's mind that day. At first, the swim was a brawl. Competitors jockeyed for position with limbs becoming virtual weapons. Navigating through stroking hands and kicking feet that clipped me from all directions, I fought back and held my position while keeping a constant eye on the course markers. Closer and closer they came until I was turning around and swimming back toward the shore.

The crowd of competitors that had previously struggled for space had dissolved. In the calm water, I felt the ripple under my streamlined body as my hands curved and cut at the water. Peeking up to spot the shore and take a breath, I noticed a number of orange swim caps behind me, more than there were in front of me. Motivated, I pushed on to the finish.

Once I was close enough to the edge of the shore, I stopped swimming and started to fling myself forward using my arms. While the water resisted me and I fought against it, I saw wet suits running to the transition area where their bikes rested on racks, ready to ride off on the next leg of the triathlon. Hitting the sand at the water's end, I threw my arms around my father's and a race volunteer's shoulders and they hurried me over to the transition where Jim was waiting to begin his fourteen-mile trek.

As we crossed the timing mat, I saw the official race clock. My time of twenty minutes to complete the half-mile swim flashed across it, and I breathed a sigh of relief. I had finished in a place that was all my own; I could not help but feel a sense of accomplishment because it was not just about completing the race. It was about competing.

While my parents and Jackie congratulated and kissed me and told me how proud of me they were, I recognized that this race was not over. Fidgeting in my seat, I was surging with the competitive spirit that resided inside of me. I was antsy; if I had a foot, I would have been tapping it. I wanted Jim to be the first one in. *Where is he?* Other competitors were coming in at around forty-five minutes, but I did not see him. Finally, when he appeared in the distance, I was practically jumping out of my seat and hooting for him. After an hour and fifteen minutes, he came across the finish line in a panting hurry.

"What took you so long?" I said with a smile.

Stretching out, he grimaced and said, "It was a lot hillier than I thought it would be." Then, he told me that he did not get off of his bike and walk it at certain parts like some of the other competitors did. Instead, he had made it up all of the hills, passing people along the way who were not up to the task. "Team Tartaglio," as Jim had named us, was not about giving up.

With Jim back, Jackie was off to complete her three-mile run. I could feel the camaraderie we had among us. There were a lot of back pats that day, as we joked about what went right and what did not. Jim informed me that I was wearing a surfing wet suit. Looking down at my getup and then around at some of the other team athletes, we both laughed at my novice triathlon experience. "It's your fault!" I hollered at Jim.

As Jackie came to the finish, my first triathlon was officially over; but, it would not be my last. Congregating as a team, we congratulated one another. Team Tartaglio had placed in the middle of the pack, an effort that we had accomplished on the strength of our individual events.

This day reinforced what I already knew about myself. Surviving was a miracle in itself. I truly felt that it was by the stroke of God that I was able to find people who had the ability to work with me and provide me with the means and the knowledge to do what was considered to be impossible.

Regardless of all that I had been through, I was here now, celebrating the completion of a successful triathlon with my team.

17

Dressed in a Polo T-shirt and shorts, I wanted to make a good first impression. His office was located in the Thomas J. Walsh Athletic Center, a formidable structure, unlike the Rec Plex. Within a ranging parking lot that ran out of view, the Athletic Center was flanked by a turf field on the left and fenced-in tennis courts on the right. After opening the door to the complex, I followed the sound of clanking weights to a corridor. As I got closer to the end of the whitewashed hallway, my nose began to track the scent of sweat.

When I pushed into a weight room about the size of an aircraft hangar, there were a few people working out across the gym; but they did not seem to notice me, probably because the eclectic mix machines towered over my smaller stature.

Scheduled to meet with Head Strength and Conditioning Coach Mark Spellman about the possibility of using the Athletic Center, all I wanted was the opportunity to exercise. While I thought that Fairfield should be ashamed for letting their fitness center fall into disrepair, the condition of the "Rec Plex" was not my fight. Instead, accessibility was.

As I stared at the display of weight racks, "Coach," as the athletes called him, greeted me from his office. He was tall man in his midthirties with a cleanly shaved head. Weighing in at roughly six feet one, 220 pounds, he was not a body builder, but he held a muscular frame from years of work. Spellman was someone who was strong before he was big; his job was to instill a no-quit mentality in the athletes that he trained, so his endurance was exceptional. As he held out his hand, I shook it and he invited me in.

His countenance told me that he was not expecting someone quite like me. It was evident that Disability Services had not explained the intricacy of my situation.

"If you don't mind me asking," he said. "What happened to you?" This was a complete stranger, yet I divulged details of my situation to him as openly as if he was a family member. I considered myself lucky, I told him, and it had nothing to do with living to tell my story. There were people in this world who were worse off than me, people who were affected by trauma as severe as mine, and people who did not have the means or the support to rehabilitate like I did. Not only did I have a prosthetist who cracked the prosthetic code, but I had also worked with physical therapists who enabled me to physically become myself again. My parents had built a foundation under me that could not be amputated, giving me the strength to persevere in the face of seemingly insurmountable odds. And without the teams of support I had received from all of those strangers and friends alike, I would not even be having the conversation. I was lucky not because I had *lived*, but because I was *living*.

Spellman's face twisted when I said that I was lucky. "Huh?" he screeched. He was dumbfounded, not glancing at me but through me. After all that had happened to me, most could not understand how I could ever consider myself lucky. He was clearly grappling with this question.

"All I'm asking is for the opportunity to train, that's all," I said, somewhat pleading. This was not a question of preference so much as it was necessity. The school weight room was substandard. I needed an adequate facility that I could independently access and maneuver within.

Silence sat between us. The seconds felt like minutes. With his hand on his face, he looked at me and continued to search for his response. Any hope I had to use the facility hinged on his decision.

Finally, he nodded and shrugged. "Sure, you can come in here."

"Great!" my voice cracked like a pubescent child. I was not necessarily surprised, but rather appreciative because I recognized that he did not have to grant me this permission.

"If you don't mind, I would like to bring in a partner to help me out," I nervously fumbled with my words, asking for a favor after receiving his generosity, "when it's OK with you, of course, and I'm not in the way of the teams or anyone. Everything else I can take care of myself."

He shook his head and smiled. "Don't worry about that," he said. "I'll be working with you."

He'll be working with me? I was not his responsibility. He was paid to train athletes; I was not a Fairfield University athlete, and I did not expect to have the privilege of working with him. No matter how many times I tried to graciously tell him that his help was not necessary, he simply would not have it. He was genuinely interested in helping me.

"We're going to have to schedule some time into my busy schedule," he said. "How do mornings work for you?" Jokingly, I grumbled and told him that I had a morning class, but before or after would be fine.

"Is there anything that you can't do?" he asked.

"Leg machines, but everything else I can make happen," I quipped. For me, there was no could not.

We talked about the Madison Jaycees and how I had really taken to swimming over the past year. More triathlons were in my future, but my immediate goals were direct; I wanted to get stronger and continue to build my stamina so that I could use my running leg more frequently. Conversely, Spellman shared that he had swum in college and also had experience with disabled athletes. While working in Maryland, he had trained the Achilles track team, a group of disabled athletes.

When Spellman talked about his past work with "disabled" athletes, I realized that, in every sense of the word, I was disabled. At the same time, I never felt like my predicament held me back from doing what I wanted to do. While I drove a car unlike someone who had legs, I was still driving. While my walk was atypical in look and in feel, I was still able to take steps. There were no labels that defined me.

Even after our initial meeting, I think Spellman was somewhat skeptical about me wanting to come in on my own time and work out. This was an unfamiliar scenario for him; I wasn't a groaning athlete forced to wake up early for practice. I wanted to be there, and I wanted to bust my ass.

****

I thought that I had strong workout acumen from the months that I spent with Jim and Dave, but Spellman opened my eyes to a new style of training that I had not even considered.

"Like most males, you're only interested in training your chest and your arms," Spellman joked. "I'm trying to educate you that there's more to your body than just your chest. We need to get your core, abs, and back stronger for what you want to do. Everyone wants to look good, but we need to get you prepared."

While what we were doing was not necessarily different, how we were doing it and the rate at which it was being done was. Spellman showed me alternate ways to compound exercises and do more in less time. There was little to no rest in between sets. Intensity, not time, became our focus. A shoulder workout that would generally take me a half hour to forty minutes took roughly fifteen to twenty minutes with Spellman. He would have me start a set and work me until I could barely lift the weight. Then, after he yelled some "encouragement," he would assist me to do more. Within the first few minutes of our session, I would be swimming in sweat. By the end, my muscles would simply be swimming.

****

My schedule began at 6:00 a.m. every day: train, class, schoolwork, and, if there was time, socialize. Applied calculus, freshman English, general biology, general inorganic chemistry, and two labs consumed my days and nights. The transition from high school to college was far from textbook. Whereas high school focused on the general, college studies were more detail oriented. By the time I began to grasp a topic that I had learned in high school, we were already moving on to details that made it seem like an entirely new subject.

I thought that just because I took notes in class, I knew the material. I was wrong. College was not interested in memorization; instead, I was expected to make my own meaning of the course material and then be able to apply it in real-life contexts.

****

My actions were beginning to convince Spellman that I was unlike anyone he had ever worked with before. No matter how many times he pushed me down, no matter how hard he worked me, no matter how exhausted I was, I would always come back for more. To him, it was refreshing to see someone come in and work out with no pretense and, most importantly, no complaint.

Some of the athletes would even ask him why he didn't take it easy on me. But I did not want him to, and he never did. I had something to prove to him, to myself, and I guess to everyone who I encountered in

103

the weight room. While my body was physically different from theirs, what I was doing was not.

"I treat you like an eighteen- to twenty-five-year old male college athlete—I don't give you any quarter, I don't let you get away with anything," Spellman said. "At the end of the day, I have a job to do, which is to see beyond any limitations you could have with the wheelchair. After a point, I do not even see the wheelchair."

Fairfield coaches who were in the weight room began to take notice of my dedicated effort. Many of them approached Spellman about having me talk to their respective teams as a means to motivate them. He informed me of their interest, but I did not feel ready to open myself up to strangers, especially kids my own age, about all that I had been through. Spellman, like many others, encouraged me to keep speaking in mind for the future. I had a story to tell, and apparently there were people who were interested in hearing it.

****

Among adjusting to the college workload, seeing progress with Spellman, and forging friendships in the dorm, I seemed to be finding my home in Fairfield. However, while some relationships rise, others crumble. And it ended up being my relationship with my girlfriend that fell by wayside.

We had only been dating for a year and a half, but it felt longer because of everything I had been through. She was the girl who I had called from the operating table when I thought I would never see her again. She had seen me at my lowest when not even the doctors were certain if I would survive. She had stuck by me when I asked her if she still wanted to be with someone *like* me. And now, she was gone.

When I went home to Milford for winter break, we met in person for the first time since early November. The separation had clearly taken a toll on each of us. What seemed so right no longer was. I had to accept that she no longer wanted to be with me.

She was that first breakup that really taught me life lessons. Like any other self-conscious eighteen-year-old, I wondered if there was anyone who would ever love me again. In my case, I didn't know if there were any girls who would accept me since I had no legs.

Mike was always there to remind me that life did not end with the close of a relationship. If it wasn't for him, I might have alternated between exercise and class for the rest of my college career. While I was not shy, I was not Mike either. He was a megaphone that grabbed a room's attention, a social conduit who drew others toward his charming, effervescent personality. Whether I was interacting with the people around me, making a joke, talking about that cute girl, complaining about a class, and then saying hey to that cute girl, Mike gave me the confidence to be myself.

In the midst of all of the emotions that linger after a relationship fails, I stopped by Rehabilitation Associates to see Jim. It was refreshing to see a friendly face. Catching up, we talked about how I intended to prepare for my two-mile walk at our 5K benefit run. Unlike the previous one that had raised money for my recovery, this 5K was my way of giving back to all of those who had given so much to me. Jim and I planned to award a college scholarship to a high school student who was able overcome personal adversity and achieve academic success.

Since it was not snowing over winter break, I hit the track in the walking legs. I had not worn them since before I went away to school, so I anticipated that my time in them would be torturous; yet, as I made my way around the blacktop bend, I did not experience the agony and the ache that came from wearing them. I soon realized that calluses had developed on my hips that allowed me to wield the prosthetics for longer than ever before. The motions that I had tripped over for months were no longer a concern. I did not worry about the crutch length, or how far I was swinging; those were all small details that would detract from my main purpose—moving forward.

With my newfound poise in my prosthetics, I realized that I could not rest on walking two miles. A few days before I went back to Fairfield, I paid Jim another visit.

"You know what?" I said, assuredly and not waiting for his response to my question. "I'm going to run the 5K."

As always, Jim was on board. The man who had believed in me when I did not even believe in myself had no objections. "Absolutely, you can do that!" He was as excited about it as I was. "Do you want me to walk with you during the race?"

Equally as energized, I accepted Jim's offer. He would be there to push me, pace me, and pick me up, just as he had always done.

The breakup with my girlfriend was heartbreaking. I did not know if any other girl would accept me for who I was. While I realized that we were not right for each other, I also knew that some females had a tough time looking past my disability. While I tried to play it cool, I could not help feeling self-conscious. There were enough guys out there who had similar qualities as me but had legs too. How would I ever stack up against them?

It was not until a few months after our breakup that I was able to answer that question. It was as if a light went off in my head—an epiphany of sorts. While I might have shared common traits with other guys, they were certainly not the same. No one else had experienced exactly what I had and come out of it the way I did. I stopped thinking that there was no one else who wanted to be with me and realized what I had to offer to someone else. Taking pride in who I was for the first time, I began to move forward, learn from my mistakes, and have better relationships. By acknowledging my value and realizing the way that I could enrich peoples' lives by interacting with them, it helped me gain self-worth.

This positive perception helped me find the woman I am in love with and happily married to today. Once you find the person who you truly love, never take them for granted. Appreciate them for who they are and the happiness they bring you. If you treat them with this in mind, you will never go wrong. Finding happiness and fulfillment comes when you can look at yourself and your actions and believe in who you are and what you are doing.

18

Whereas a year ago walking two miles was a lofty goal, now, in comparison to what I was aiming for, it seemed pedestrian.

In the beginning of February, I received a letter from Erik's office inviting me to compete in the ASPIRE 10K road race as a member of Team A Step Ahead. So a mere two weeks before the benefit I would be running half of the ASPIRE, and although I viewed the ASPIRE as a warm-up, I still had my pride. Not only did I owe it to Erik and my team to have a good showing, but I also owed it to myself; for me, there was no last place.

In my second semester, I began to wear my prosthetics on a daily basis. While I walked around in them, the prohibitive winter months made it difficult to train outside. Even when I could, the running legs were not an option; once strapped in, I could not sit down or even take my hands off of the crutches to get a drink. Asking someone to follow me around the track like a service dog was not practical nor was shuttling back to Milford so my parents could help me.

The only solution appeared to be training in the walking prosthetics instead, doing slightly less mileage in the heavier prosthetics while still incrementally increasing my distance around the track. Having limited practice in the running legs, notwithstanding, my hips were conditioned to the unforgiving scrapes and scars that the device left, and I could push myself without having to manage the accompanying pain. I did not doubt that I would be able to complete the race.

****

The sun, a sunny side-up egg on the edge of the sky, warmed my face as I watched my vaporous breath dissipate in front of me. At seven in the morning on Sunday, with the dew sitting untouched on the grass, I was at Madeline Middle School in Plainview, Long Island.

This was not an exclusively "disabled" event; anyone could participate to raise money for the New York-based nonprofit group ASPIRE, which provided children and young adults with limb loss the chance to lead healthy, active, everyday lives. It was fitting that Team A Step Ahead was involved in this function. Erik had built his business on the belief that his patients "live life without limitations."

Outside of our team, there were a handful of disabled athletes competing that day; however, the majority of the approximately three hundred people who were running the race were "able-bodied." I was the only bilateral hip disarticulate there. I had not thought about it up until that point, but I would be the first ever to run a 5K. *First ever*, the words repeated in my head. If I could pull this off, it would be the first time in history that someone without legs had ever run a 5K.

With my mind moving faster than my legs, the race was about to begin. Dave was there with me. Showing off his late-fifties man legs in his short-shorts, he would keep me hydrated while my parents would be by my side throughout the run. Since I was not starting the race from the beginning, we drove to the 5K mark. From there, I would go off about thirty minutes before the pack so I could finish with them.

Strapped in and standing up, I leaned against the car and looked around the residential area. It was a straight road with trees and modest-size houses stretching across both sides. *At least the ground is flat.* My initial thought was insignificant, though; once I was out there, I could not predict what terrain I would encounter.

If I didn't get moving soon, I might jump out of my prosthetics. I just needed the race to start. And with the sign from Dave, it did.

From my hands, up through my arms, and into my shoulders, I absorbed the road's fury and unleashed my retort, springing forward like a pole-vaulter. More than ever before, I trusted the running legs, as the clank of the carbon fiber against the pavement was quickening with each stride.

Although speed was at the forefront of my mind, I was also conscious that the flat ground I was chugging along had begun to arch up, the precursor to an upcoming downhill. And there it was, like a dipping roller coaster dropping from its highest peak. Soon, the houses became farther and farther apart and the road widened; dilapidated log fences intermittently announced a property line here and there until eventually the fences stopped, the houses hid, and a wooded area consumed my surroundings.

The road was dusty now. For a time a tumbleweed could have blown over and it would not have looked out of place on this desolate path, but we were no longer alone. At first, it was only a handful of them, men and women who would be completing the 10K in a little over a half hour. Then, like a school of fish, the masses began to swarm. Packed together in bunches, runners zipped by me. Many wished me luck as they pushed past us, but I was so focused on the path ahead of me that I did not offer them more than the occasional head nod.

In the distance, I could hear cars. Closer and closer the sounds came, yet I could not see them. When the ground leveled out, I found civilization again where signs warned the runners to proceed with caution. While a cop was assisting us in crossing the street, the four-lane road was not blocked off. As cars slowed, passengers stared for a second at the spectacle that was the runners streaming past them.

This was no longer a residential block but rather a corporate section of the town where indiscernible business buildings bunched together like boxes stacked on a shelf. For a moment, the road granted me a reprieve of a flat quarter mile. But it was only for a moment before the sun stood on my head and I made the turn to ascend a climbing hill.

My sweat-smattered face denoted the exhaustion that was trying to hijack my body. Digging the crutches into the ground, I pushed myself into each grueling step and felt the friction ignite my enflamed hands. I could only hope *I will do this* the end of the race *I will do this* was near.

Turning off of the downhill, I could see the other runners ahead of me crossing the finish line. Still, footsteps crept close behind—my competition. *Last was not, and would never be, an option.* It was within reach. "Push it through the finish, young man!" Dave barked in my ear.

There were no thoughts, simply motions ingrained for moments like this when will takes over the body. "Coming in is number one sixty-two," the race emcee called out as I approached the end. "Let's give it up for John Tartaglio!" One more flail before I broke the plane of the finish line and was smothered with love by my parents.

Joyfully exhausted, I was satisfied, not because I was able to accomplish the race, but because it was a further reminder that I could do more. Although it took me an hour and twenty-five minutes to do 3.1 miles, compared to the fifty minutes that it had taken me to do a quarter of a mile at last year's benefit, I wanted to go faster.

However, like any fight worth fighting, I needed to recover. My once steely shoulders slouched under the strain of the heavy, rope-like arms that hung from them. Meanwhile, the running legs that I had finally believed in had bludgeoned my hips callously.

Looking down at my medium-rare hands, however, I knew that I would not have asked for anything else. I had gone up against the odds, and I had won. It was not lost on me that, if I wanted to continue to compete, I had to work twice as hard as the next guy. And I would. *And I would.*

19

The weather forecast was reminiscent of the New Testament. Forget about ominous or foreboding, the sky was intimidating. Woken up by the rain punching at my window, I looked out to see grass wilting against the relentless wind and patches of puddles crashing like waves against the walkway. We had a race to run.

While the light had prevailed through the darkness at last year's benefit, it was clear that day was not today. The crowds were not swarming when I pulled up to Foran High. Apparently and justifiably, many people thought that the event was canceled; however, with all of the volunteers and the police scheduled for the day and participants beginning to show up, it was too late to call the event. Besides, we had scholarships to give out.

Standing in my running leg alongside Jim and my mother, my saturated shorts hung from my hips. While I tried to concentrate on the competition, there was none. The benefit was friendly; nobody was fighting for position like the run to the water in the triathlon.

Jim not only was my race partner that day, but he was also my pants partner as well. Because of the downpour, my shorts slipped lower and lower until they were down to the floor. Jim had to, on multiple occasions, pull them back to their rightful place. No matter how tight he tied them, they would not stay up. A padlock could not have kept those shorts around my waist that day. After some frustration, I was able to laugh with Jim and my mother. Together, we navigated through the flooded streets, as sewers gurgled and islands formed within the ocean-sized puddles.

Even though we had fewer runners than we had expected, we were still able to raise enough money to award two scholarships to ease the cost of college. I was not even sure who won the race, but it did not matter. This day was not about winning and losing or competitive showings; instead, it was about giving back to the community that had given so much to me. I would never forget how they enabled me to lead a normal, functional life.

Following the momentum of my swinging athletic ambitions, I began to consider a possibility that I had brushed aside in the past. The idea of motivational speaking was first presented to me within a month of my stay in the hospital. At the time, I had discounted the suggestion as nothing more than a nice compliment. The pain was far too recent to share with strangers. Later, after I met Spellman, he, like those who had visited me in the hospital, again suggested motivational speaking as a potential opportunity that I should pursue. Yet I did not think that I had accomplished anything worth speaking to a crowd about.

Despite my misgivings, I accepted an invitation to speak with Jim at a middle school in Orange, CT, in late April. This would mark the first time I recounted my story before an actual audience. I was there, alongside real-life heroes like fire fighters and police officers. I was nervous; I had never done this before, and I had no idea what to say to these kids. Since I did not prepare a speech, the only comfort I had was that Jim was there with me.

For five minutes, I dragged my feet through a plodding, uninspired account. I made my remarkable trek against seemingly insurmountable odds seem more like a nightly news report. There was simply the then and the now. With Jim's help, I made it through the first session, and as I spoke to other classes, I started to focus on a certain underlying point that I wanted to relay to the students: regardless of the odds, they cannot quit.

While I recognized that my public speaking skills needed some polishing, I could only hope that the kids took as much from the experience as I did. They must have because a few days later the teacher told me how much everyone enjoyed me, and I was encouraged to come back next year.

The circumstances of my situation were as tragic as they were inspiring. What I had done, what I was doing, and what I would continue to do, was a moving, constantly evolving story. Although my predicament was atypical, I could draw life lessons from my experiences that others could relate to. Maybe it was time to tell my story to help people live better lives.

Within a month of being in the hospital, people told me that I should be a motivational speaker. Each time I heard it, I thought it was such a nice compliment, but I did not see the purpose in it. I did not think I had accomplished anything worth speaking to crowds about. At that time, it was too early for me to consider speaking to others about what had happened to me. It was not that I was uncomfortable; I just did not know the first thing about presenting my story to a crowd.

By the beginning of college, as I started to get back to a normal regimen, I gave speaking more thought. My debut at the middle school near my house was a breakthrough in my speaking career. I realized that I stunk, but after a few shots at telling my story to the rotating classrooms of kids, I became a better storyteller. And it hit me that day—just by spending a few minutes speaking to the children, I was able to connect with them. They were attentively listening to my story and to me.

The whole point of being a speaker is to affect the crowd in one way or another. Whether I had inspired new hope for the future in a teary-eyed woman recently released from the hospital or given a well-respected businessman a new perspective not only to appreciate what he had but also to be a better leader, I was humbled. If I could help one person with my story in any way, then speaking was worth much more than any compensation I would receive.

20

"Have you ever given any thought to hand cycling in the New York City Marathon?"

There was a pause. The words of the hand-cycling retailer Bike-On's representative lingered on the other end of the line imploring me to say something, anything. *What excuse is there? I'm new to this game, so I don't know that a hand-cycle division exists?*

In a moment of abashed ignorance, I laughed awkwardly and quickly replied, "No." *But why not? Why couldn't I do it?*

Since the Madison Jaycees, I had wanted to compete in an entire triathlon—not just swimming but cycling and running too. At that point in my life, though, still limited by the running prosthetics and the intensive training they required, I began to think why not hand cycle the New York City Marathon instead? My plans were about to change.

****

By chance, I received a letter from Gaylord inviting me to a hand cycling clinic where I met with a Bike-On technician in person and tested out a base model hand cycle.

With two wheels in the back and one in the front and pedals where handlebars would be, it was like a tricycle for disabled adults. Although my hands and arms acted as feet and legs did for a cyclist, the exercise of keeping the bike moving seemed simple enough. How wrong I was.

Cranking away at the pedals as if I was competing against them, I was losing. As other bikers passed me by, the wheels still spun, around and around, circling, spinning, moving, everyone and everything but me. It seemed that even the road was outracing me that day. Still, with my shoulders sizzling and my stamina suffocating, knowing then that there was nothing 'simple' about it, I walked out of the expo with a hand cycle and the intention of riding the New York City Marathon as well.

****

Set for the first Sunday in November, the marathon was upon me. It was already almost August, and with only three months to prepare for the 26.2-mile race, Erik still had to outfit the bike with a custom seat. Waiting and losing time on the hand cycle I had only ridden once, I should have been feeling the pressure. Yet I was not. Everything seemed to be falling into place once Dave agreed to train me. All I had to do was start riding, and I would be ready for November 7.

Then, reality set in. My magnificent marathon plan would have to wait until next year. The deadline to sign up had passed. Could an exception be made? Not for me. Maybe if I was someone else, someone more important. *Maybe if I had signed up on time, I would not have had to worry about it.* Was there anyone who could help me? *Dave. He had to know somebody.* As it turned out, he did, and he contacted Amy Palermo-Winters—a below-the-knee amputee who was an avid, accomplished runner and a member of Team A Step Ahead. Using her connections, she helped me secure a spot in the race. I would be riding in New York City after all.

****

Dave tried to put hand cycling in perspective for me when we were practicing one day in Central Park. He pointed out the obvious; legs have more muscles than arms, so I couldn't exert the power or exhibit the speed of a cyclist. For this reason, the best cyclist would always beat the best hand cyclist. The design of the hand cycle, in general, did not help my cause either. Having an additional wheel on my bike meant that there was extra friction I had to overcome. A little more work to do an activity

120

like an able-bodied person was nothing new to me. I had gotten used to it as the price of doing business when you're amputated up to your hipbones.

With the sun bearing down on me like a foot on my back, I began to ride around. At first, the motion was manageable and I enjoyed the exercise. Turning. Whirling. Central Park was much hillier than I remembered. Twisting. Wrenching. Then, the foot grew heavier. Twirling. Writhing. And its kick became cruel. Craned over in the same aerodynamic position for hours, my back felt like there was a vice clamping down on it.

Six miles later, I looked over to Dave in disbelief. *What have I gotten myself into?* Transferring into my wheelchair and immediately slouching over, I tried to dispel my doubts about the marathon. Muscles I did not even know existed were twitching so hard that I wondered if they had broken the skin. My back felt like a flabby belly. While I did not expect to be Lance Armstrong my first day out there, I never could have imagined that my introduction to cycling would leave me questioning if I ever wanted to do it again.

****

Erik had to be able to do something, offer some suggestion to get me back on track. He always had a solution.

"Couldn't you put a pad on there or something [to lean my chest against], at least so I can rest my back?"

I could see his head shaking over the phone before he answered me. "Over the course of a race, it's just not practical. It'll put too much pressure on your chest and end up restricting you." Essentially, if this was a goal that I wanted to pursue, I needed to suck it up and do it.

Once I returned to Fairfield for my sophomore year, roughly two months before the marathon, I did not know when I would find time to train. Because school always came first, I was not able to put in the consecutive hours on the bike that I needed to. Instead, I had to break up the miles over the course of the day between morning and afternoon sessions. Luckily, Spellman was generous enough to let me keep my bike on a stationary track stand in the athletic center.

Like my mindset heading into the Madison Jaycees, hand cycling the marathon was not just about being there. I wanted to compete. Every day was a new test of my endurance. Up before some of my peers walked in the door, I would be on the bike by 6:00 a.m. After about an hour and a half, I would get into it with Spellman. From presses to flies to dips, the weight was more manageable than the pace where seconds—not minutes—were taken in between sets. I felt as if I was more sweat than body. And it felt good.

Maybe it was wishful thinking and maybe my confidence was giving me false hope, but one day after a workout I told Spellman that I wanted to finish in the top twenty. No matter how unrealistic it actually was, I still thought it was plausible. He, however, reeled in my expectations and reminded me that just completing the race was an accomplishment.

"I don't doubt you—I never do—but I don't want you to feel let down if you don't do it," he said. "Why not top thirty?"

****

By October, I had accumulated twenty-four total miles over the course of a day. However, there would be no afternoon siesta in the middle of the New York City Marathon. So in the remaining weeks leading up to the marathon, I returned to Milford on the weekends to put together consecutive miles. Up until that point, I had not done more than sixteen miles on the road.

One morning, on the road just as the sun was getting out of bed, I took a deep breath. Having mapped out the distance of my trek, I knew how many times that I had to go around the back roads surrounding my house in order to hit my mark of twenty-four miles. This was it, the longest distance I had attempted in succession. I was confident, but was I ready? I would soon find out.

Zipping down the street like a Matchbox car on a track, I was no longer laboring with each turn of the pedal. I had a rhythm, a motion that I had not had when I worked with Dave in Central Park. Revolution after revolution, the wheels hypnotically spun as I passed through neighboring streets and the miles whittled away.

When I pulled up at an indiscriminant location that was the figurative finish line, I eagerly looked at my shaking arm for my time. Seeing the numbers and registering them in my head—*two and a half hours? TWO AND A HALF HOURS!*—I wished I hadn't even looked. All of my vitality dissipated from my body like a deflated balloon. If I could've stayed in that spot all day, I might have. How did I expect to finish in the top twenty when that number would have put me near the back of the pack? *This was my last chance to prove myself, and I blew it.*

With a little over two weeks before the race, I had to begin to scale back my miles. I was caught in a catch-22; I did not want a lack of stamina to hold me back from fulfilling my goal, but I needed to conserve my energy for the race. So many questions were still unanswered, but as my hourglass dwindled, my time had just about run out.

21

I could not sleep; the silent solitude of the dark, dead night danced around the room. I was hot. Then the pillow wasn't cold. I tossed and turned through the sheets as the city lights cast shadows against the walls, taunting my efforts to sleep.

"On your MARK!" The words rang through my head like a shot fired, and then I opened my eyes. The phone was ringing for my 5:00 a.m. wake-up call. I quickly hopped out of bed and hurriedly readied myself to catch a bus with the rest of the cyclists and wheelers, or racers using push rim-racing wheelchairs.

We were being transported over to the starting point of the race, right before the Verrazano-Narrows Bridge in Staten Island. Looking around, I was by far the youngest person there. When we arrived I forced myself to have a half of a bagel, but my stomach, filled with the anticipation of what I had been preparing for for three strenuous months, was revolting against me.

At 7:15 a.m., the wheelers began their trek. Then, minutes before 7:30 a.m., the hand cyclers gained access to the bridge and starting line. I was toward the back of the swell.

Along the sidelines, a race director raised the megaphone to his mouth. Eyes were fixated on him as every one of the competitors took a position. There was a pause with the anticipation of what would come next. "Go!" he shouted, and we were off like horses out of the gate. Some of the group remained toward the back as they tried to pace themselves. With about a hundred people jockeying to set themselves apart from the rest, I refused to stay in my position near the end of the group. I did not come to New York to finish last. Instead, I began making my move early on.

We were going over the Verrazano with our wheels clicking against the grates like a typewriter resetting at the end of a line. While I tried to compare myself to the competitors who surrounded me in that first mile of the race, I was passing them and picking up confidence with each turn of the wheel. I no longer felt like I was throwing my back out with each turn. This was my confirmation that my training had prepared me for the race.

As the wind was picking up from the water and the sun was just beginning to break through the overcast sky, I rattled off of the Verrazano, past a park, and onto Ninety-Fifth Street into Brooklyn. Perusing the passing storefronts, an ever-changing collection of ethnic eateries, I breathed in the smells of the neighborhoods. Chinese, Italian, Polish, Indian, Vietnamese, Middle Eastern, there was something for even the most particular of eaters. Everywhere I turned, I saw a different face, smiling, waving, and cheering me on.

Past the Brooklyn brownstones and the flashing lights of police escorts, we wheeled through streets like we owned them. The city was still the city around us, but Fourth Avenue was ours that day. There was no shortage of spectators as we turned onto Lafayette Avenue; with music playing and the crowd roaring, they offered support that willed us around each bend and up every hill. It was like a block party that did not stop at the end of the block.

There was some organization to where the spectators were situated, besides the barricades and police presence. Similar to the ASPIRE 10K, the largest crowds were situated near the most trying portions of the marathon to give the competitors an emotional boost. It certainly helped having people scream encouraging words in your direction. I could only imagine how professional athletes felt during a game.

In Queens, the streets lost their names, the rivers became one, and the band played on to the beat of the spinning wheels. We proceeded over a bridge called Pulaski; I had never heard of it, and I would not have been able to identify it if I was driving over it. Compared to the up and down climb of the Verrazano, it felt more like a speed bump. However, after a few blocks where I could have been flying, there was a sharp turn onto Queens Boulevard leading up to the Queensboro Bridge. This was the sixteen-mile mark, but I was not slouched, and I was not huffing when I reached it. I had my metaphorical legs under me, and to my surprise, my pace had not slowed down. I would trudge on, into Manhattan and onto First Avenue with the same burst I had from the start.

By this point the crowds were buzzing, imploring us to keep going, past the mini-marts, the furniture shops, and the kosher delis. But there was no doubt in my mind that I would finish strongly; that was an end I knew I would meet. I was thinking about my talk with Spellman and the goal that we had set, thirtieth place, repeating it in my head after each person I passed along the way.

As I made it through the Bronx, over the rickety Willis Avenue Bridge that felt like it was going to collapse and into Manhattan, the race was drawing closer to its conclusion. The buildings rose higher and higher, apartments and offices alike competing for the sky's attention. Around the twenty-two-mile mark, I began to feel a tired tension in my shoulders. They were as heavy as sandbags around my neck. I could have hit the wall, I could have taken a breather, I could have given up, but I did not climb this mountain to turn back around. This was the peak that I had trained for. I was almost to the top, and there was nothing that could have stopped me from getting there.

Another competitor was ahead of me. We were climbing a hill, the highest and most strenuous yet. My adrenaline was pumping. The crowds were scattered along the sidelines to the top where I could see the ground level out. Hands clapped and mouths yelled; but, in that moment, it was only him and me.

Closer and closer I came, his back strained and his shoulders bulging. Putting hand to wheel, I maneuvered around him and took my place ahead of him. We weaved back and forth, neither of us trying to concede our position. He did not want to lose any more ground, but I would not relinquish mine. It was chess on wheels: who would hold out the longest and who would be held in check. And all the while, the crowd did not relent.

Through Central Park we went with the finish line coming into view and my competition at my back. Waiving my arms up and down to spur on the spectators, they obliged and boomed praise on us as they had done all day.

When I crossed the finish line, my supporters smothered me. With a blanket draped over me and with my closest friends and family by my side, I basked in the accomplishment of what I had just done. After only a few months of training, I had bested the 26.2-mile event and earned my place that day.

"John!" a voice that I did not recognize called to me through my blockade of friends and family. It was a journalist, ready to take notes with his pad in hand. "How do you feel?"

"I feel really good," I said. "It was a lot easier than I thought." His face twisted in disbelief and he let out an awkward laugh to sugarcoat his surprise, but I was serious. Coming in at 2:12:12, I had bested my disenchanting 24-mile time from my marathon tune-up. And did I have a story for Spellman. I had finished in thirtieth place!

The first time I walked the quarter of a mile around the track, my competitive mentality returned to me. Even though I loved team sports, the way endurance events allowed me to push myself was a perfect match.

I started from the shorter distance road races and triathlons, competing in a 5K and sprint triathlon first. But I wanted more. The 10K, individual sprint triathlons, and Olympic and half ironmans were next.

The only way to break through boundaries and push past your limits is by having a vision. You can't expect to be successful without a goal in mind. And no target is any good without a plan. You need a personal road map so you can hold yourself accountable to execute the steps necessary to meet your goals.

22

"July 13. Providence, Rhode Island. Swim. Bike. Run. Seventy point three miles. You in?"

His answer was almost subconscious. Without hesitation, he said, "Where do I sign up?" There was no need to question Chris's word. He was paying his own way through college and had been living on his own since he was eighteen. I knew that I could rely on him.

The Amica half ironman, which consisted of a 1.2-mile swim, a 56-mile bike ride, and a 13.1-mile run, would be the most physically demanding competition I had ever participated in. While the race coordinator, in her concerned, parental tone, had cautioned me that the bike portion was "hilly," she could not dissuade me from registering. I might have been the only disabled athlete signed up for the event, but I was still a competitor.

****

By the third week in January, my second semester junior year, my focus shifted to the ASPIRE 10K. Unlike the previous year where I ran the 5K portion of the race, I looked to push myself further and run the entire 6.2 miles from start to finish.

To accomplish this goal, I had branched out and picked up a new training partner in Brett Hunchak. A friend of mine since freshman year, he had always kept in shape more so for the aesthetics of it than the health benefits. However, it was not until junior year that he had committed to his fitness and to me.

Whether it was a spot or a countdown, Brett helped me on a day-to-day basis where Spellman could not. Some days we would do less, others we would do more, but the exercises were extensions of what I was doing with Spellman. There was no quit; there was no stop. It was go, always.

Alternating between workout sessions with Spellman and Brett on a daily basis, I tried to build my stamina up even faster than when I cycled the New York City Marathon. Yet no matter how many weights I lifted or how many laps I swam, there was no substitute to getting out to the track. That presented a problem for me since someone had to walk with me in case I needed a drink or, worse, if I fell. Training in the running leg was not an option, so I decided to use the walking leg instead. In a prosthetic that was ten pounds heavier than the running leg and with a twenty-pound weight vest strapped to my back, I trudged around the track reasoning that the extra weight would compensate for my lack of miles.

However, time was competing against me. Less than two weeks remained before the ASPIRE. The 1.5 miles I was walking did not come close to the 6.2 miles I would be required to run. While I hoped that I was physically prepared for what I was about to do, faith did not change fact. I was not ready for that imminent Sunday.

23

It was the same Madeline Middle School as it was the year before. While the course had not changed, I had never seen the first half of it. For the first time in months, there I stood in my running legs. *When I cross the finish line, I will be the only person without legs to ever complete a 10K.* I could only hope that my alternative training regimen would allow me to be competitive.

I hung my head and waited for Dave's voice. Again, I would be starting before the rest of the field so I could finish with them. In that instance, as the sun stroked my hair, the green, growing world around me was abuzz with spring. The ASPIRE always seemed to have optimal weather unlike the benefits that Jim and I put on. Thinking back to the last benefit, it was so windy that I could not even keep my pants up. A smile crept across my face.

"Let's go!" Dave yelled, signaling the informal start of my race. Light on my waist, the running leg easily curled forward with the crutches firmly placed against the ground, the flex foot hitting, and me swinging into my next step.

Through the street I went, as the red sun began to rise overhead and the houses grew farther apart. Flawless white plastic fences gave way to rustic wooden log dividers. Looking for a course marker to point me in the right direction, my parents picked up the sign from the race map and instructed me to turn right. Up a hill we went, and no amount of weight on my back could have prepared me for that climb. Winded like my lungs were holding their breath, I could feel the incline. I knew I should have ratcheted up my endurance training, but in that moment, what did it matter?

Looking around, I no longer saw any indicators of where the next leg of the race was. My parents were dumbfounded. *Had we taken a wrong turn? Where were we?* I had already gone about a quarter of a mile. Did I turn around and go back to the cross street, or should I keep going and see where this takes me? The questions darted around my head like points on an indiscernible road map. We were lost.

"Don't worry," my parents tried to assuage my concerns, "everything will be fine. We'll turn around and get back on the course. Just keep going and finish the race."

An inexplicable amount of curses were muttered at this time. I wanted to scream, but there was no explanation for what had happened and pointing fingers would not get me to the finish any faster. This event suddenly felt like a waste of time. Trudging along with no particular path, my mind was on autopilot. My muscles were reacting, but I had lost the nerve to compete. When we found the course marker and tried to make up ground, by that point the 10K had already won.

Rounding the turn onto the straightaway, I soon saw Madeline Middle School come into focus. Unlike the previous year when cheering spectators lined the sidewalks, the galleries were empty now. The water stations were being packed up, and, while my parents were there to encourage me to the finish, I was alone on that deserted road.

When I crossed the finish line as the first bilateral hip disarticulate to ever complete a 10K run, the race emcee did not even announce me coming in; there was nobody to tell. An accomplishment had never felt so disheartening. The awards ceremony was wrapping up, and only a handful of people remained to see my walk of shame. Erik, along with members of Team A Step Ahead, congratulated me, but there was no amount of praise that would ease my mind. I had failed; it took me over three hours to finish an event that should have taken me a little over two. Moving past this day was my only thought; I wanted to erase the memory of my poorest athletic showing ever. There was no achievement to hang my hat on, no pat on the back that could put this letdown in a positive light. I had never experienced such failure.

The ASPIRE 10K was supposed to be a groundbreaking day for my racing career; instead, it turned out to just be embarrassing. I would not forget coming into an empty finish line, spectators completely gone, award ceremony finished.

I had signed up for the race with an expectation to finish well, and I had broken that promise. It was a poor reflection on who I was and what I expected of myself, and I vowed that I would not put myself in that position again.

From that day alone, I learned just as much as I had any other time that I hit my expected mark. At the time, I was overwhelmed with my college workload and did not train properly. Grades always took precedence over any race. Competing was fun, it was sport, but it was not my livelihood.

There was a tangible value in academics—doing well in school meant that my future goals could be met. This, not the one race, would allow me to pursue a career that fulfilled me. Only then would I have the opportunity to live what I considered a successful life.

24

"I heard you don't have lips," a young boy no older than ten said to me. I smiled at him and his childish naivety. He meant to say limbs, but it did not matter. I knew what he was saying even if he didn't.

Toward the end of April, I had been contacted by the Darien school district. They informed me that they were holding a Jog-A-Thon at Royal Middle School and they wanted to donate the proceeds from it to help pay for part of my push rim wheelchair. I planned to use it in place of my prosthetics during the running portion of triathlons. Local elementary school children would be participating in the event, and individuals and businesses would sponsor the laps that they ran. In another instance where generosity was granted to me, I would never forget that I was able to lead an everyday life next to the guy with legs because of the anonymous support that I received.

As I sat there in the cafeteria, the children surrounded me like birds around bread, chirping away. They asked me questions about what had happened to me and how it was to be on TV. To them, I was famous, a larger-than-life figure at their school. Their teachers had explained my situation to them, but if some of the leading doctors in the country did not understand what I had been through, there was only so much a child could comprehend.

We walked outside to the field where four fluorescent orange cones were set up marking the parameters of the course. I felt like I was back at my elementary school's field day, as hundreds of pure, impressionable, baby-faced kids ran for me. This was just fun and games for them; they could not grasp what this meant to me. I had dealt with a situation that no one should ever have to go through, and I had grown up much earlier than most seventeen-year-olds did; now, at Royal Middle School, these children were giving me another opportunity to further my independence. As I saw their faces—the joy in their eyes and the playfulness in their laughs—I was a kid again.

****

Between the Pat Griskus Triathlon and the Amica half ironman that followed it, there were only a few months separating the two. When I returned to Milford for summer vacation, Chris and I began training immediately for the coming races. He was as excited as I was. Amica would be his first triathlon, let alone a half ironman. He wanted to prove to himself that he could extend himself past the realm of swimming and into the endurance athlete category.

A triathlon presented the participant with a unique dilemma. While there had to be a focus on the event that was most lacking, at the same time preparations needed to be made for the other parts of the race as well.

To acclimate myself to the physically depleting task of competing in the three separate yet interconnected events, I began to "brick train," or take two legs of the race and do them back to back. Since swimming was my most formidable leg of the race, I set out on the neighborhood focused on the other two events. After roughly fifteen miles on the hand cycle, I would hop into the push rim and head out for a four-mile spin.

Like men on a mission from a higher calling, Chris and I continued our torrid routine in the gym. We used Spellman's nonstop plan of attacking the weights with no more than thirty seconds in between sets as a guideline. As Lil Wayne wheezed, "I can see the end and the beginnin'/ So I'm not racin'/ I'm just sprintin'/ Cause I don't wanna finish / They diminish / I replenish" in my ears, eighty-pound dumbbells were pushed up and down, up and down, five times, exhaling, red-faced, arms twitching, before a twenty-second rest was taken. Ten sets and five minutes later, we had done fifty reps. With the focus on growing stamina, not muscle mass, our workouts were not about impressing anybody; they were about showing up on race day.

****

Unbeknownst to me, the Griskus had added significance to me as an amputee. Griskus was an above-the-knee amputee who had competed in triathlons and marathons across the United States and Canada in the late 1970s and 1980s. He had made history as the only amputee to complete the Hawaii Ironman in 1985 and 1986. The triathlon was named in his honor after he was hit and killed by a truck in October of 1987 while he was training for Hawaii.

My showing in the Griskus was not as important as the purpose it would serve me in my preparation for the Amica half ironman. It would be an indicator of where I was in my training. And where I was not.

****

The swim started out much the same as they all did, with the horn sounding and the competitors, both stallions and mares, galloping into the water as I swung myself behind. Expectedly, this leg of the race was not trying. However, the twenty-five-mile ride made up for any ease I had with the swim. Like a wooden roller coaster, the path climbed steep as steeple inclines followed by darting declines. As I grinded along the paved road encased by fences, fields, and foliage, my arms turned into the metal gears. Many competitors who rode beside me lauded my effort in attempting to complete the course using only my arms. My mind, however, was focused on the hilly competition that the Griskus was preparing me for. Amica would be worse, and I knew it.

When I transferred out of cycle and into the push rim, my shoulders were beaten and slumping from the hills that had battered them. This was the first time that I was using the push rim in competition, and after only a month of practice, I would soon find out if I could control it.

Darting down that first hill, the push rim sped off, leaving my stomach behind. With the wind pelting my face, I felt the speed that I could get on the hand cycle. Then, it was faster. Uncontrollably faster. My unstable body jumped from the seat. I was in the foremost fast-forward but was frantically trying to get back to play.

While I tried to use my hands to slow the wheels, they had become jet turbines, and my attempt yielded little effect. I was losing control—if I ever had it from the start. So with no time to think about the possibility of a crash or even entertain the idea of bailing out, I reacted instinctively.

"Get out of the way!" I screamed at the cone-like racers I was weaving in and out of. Luckily, they parted like street crossers do when a mad taxi is barreling toward them in New York City. Terrified, I could not imagine how they felt.

When I hit flat ground with my wheels and not my face, I was relieved to say the least. Shedding my momentum off the hill and beginning to slow down, the road stayed steady then before gradually turning me around in the direction I had come from. Keeping pace with my fellow competitors, I began to ascend the hill that had tried to kill me. While my body bore the added strain of it, my heart was at ease en route to the finish with my arms raised in triumph.

Having taken me a little under three hours to complete the Griskus, I was confident that in less than a month, I would again be riding with my arms over my head even if they were so tired that I could not feel them. However, I realized just how close I had come to catastrophe. I might not be so lucky next time.

25

Ten, the race director cleared her throat.

Nine, the faint music blared in the distance.

Eight, the muscles clapped all around.

Seven, the water chopped against the shore.

Six, the last pleasantries were exchanged.

Five, the seagulls circled overhead.

Four, the buoy pulled on its mooring.

Three, the stretches finished their exercise.

Two, the smiles no longer remained.

One.

As the pros ran past me, I pushed myself into the polar bear-cold water, crashed through a wave, and went right into my stroke. Pulling water under me and fighting off the competition, I kept my eye on the buoy and made sure that I didn't drift too far off course. When I came to the shore 1.2 miles later, my father and my uncle rushed to hoist me up.

"Hurry up!" I playfully commanded them as we crossed the electronic mat and my official time registered. With fifty-six miles to go before I reached the Providence town square, I hopped onto my bike to begin the next leg of the race.

The race director was not kidding when she told me that the terrain was hilly. Lumpy would have been a more appropriate description, as I was going up and down so much that I could have been on an elevator.

At mile twenty-six, I was scaling a hill when I looked over and there was Chris by my side.

"Hey!" he yelled hoarsely. "How ya feeling?"

In between breaths, I told him that I was good. The night before in our hotel room, we had each wanted to finish the race in less than six hours. We were on our way, he a bit quicker than me, but there was not a doubt in my mind that I could do this. There never was. He wished me luck, and, in the same instance, charged past the mass of cyclists.

Some cyclists were coasting by me, their legs churning seemingly with ease as my arms labored through each turn. But I continued on, fighting for each mile that passed, going even as my muscles ached and pleaded for a break from the continuous movement.

With only a few more miles to ride, I was coming closer to the conclusion. After passing the mile fifty-two marker at the top of one of the higher peaks I had climbed, I began to free-fall down the hill. Faster and faster I went, as my eyes strained against the rolling scenery and the wind rattled in my ears. To the left, I noticed there was a turn coming. I never saw the pothole until I was about to hit it. Violently I swerved, but my back left tire could not get out of the way and it clipped a divot. Launched into the air, I was caught, helplessly suspended in time, as the cars passed by on the other side of the road and I was thrown from the hand cycle. *SMACK!* My helmet hit the ground first, and I was rolling, taking part of the road with my shoulder, until my derriere finally brought my skidding body to a halt.

I lay there motionless for a second looking for my breath. *Is my ass broken?* The cycle, a contorted Erector Set, was in front of me; the back wheel that took the hit was detached. Dragging myself off to the side of the road, cyclists maneuvered around me. There was still a race going on, with or without me in it. As the race workers attended to me, I could hear the siren coming, closer and closer until the red lights lit ruby fires in my eyes.

While a medic cleaned the gravel out of my road-rashed shoulder, a race worker opined, "I guess you're going to have to try again next year."

My face was as stern as my simple words. "Not a chance! I didn't come this far to give up now; I'm going back out to finish."

After the mechanic reattached the wheel and bent the crooked handlebar back into place, with my shoulder slung low and the seat feeling like a bed of nails, I was off again. It was not going to be comfortable, nor would it be pretty, but I was going to complete this race if I had to crawl through the finish.

****

Pulling into the transitioning area in between events, I immediately caught my mother's frantic eyes. She had been pacing around asking the same questions, "Where is he? What's taking him so long? Have you seen my son?" One of my fellow competitors had told her that I had fallen and was being taken away in the ambulance. This really threw her into a frenzy.

"What happened? What happened?" my concerned parents asked me. No time for talk, I told them as I transferred out of the cycle and into the push rim. But my mother, being a mother, pressed me for an answer.

"I broke my ass!" I called back to her. *Was that even possible?*

As I navigated through Providence, I struggled not with the acute pain in my shoulder nor the leaden arms that compensated for it. Even my overall time didn't bother me. It was my enflamed backside that stoked my aggravation. I was constantly readjusting myself trying to find a compromise between sitting on hot coals and jagged shards of glass. Thirteen point one miles was all that separated me from an ice pack that I would sit on for the rest of my life.

While I expected the needling pain that had consumed my body to make every mile feel like two, the push rim was soaring through the streets. I even received an assist from one of the racers who started pushing me along. Although I did not want him to, I could not stop him when he got behind me; besides, it was a genuinely nice gesture, albeit telling of how some people view those with physical disabilities as needing help.

I knew that I was finally nearing the finish when I began my final ascent up a small hill that led to the end of the race. Crowds lined the sides, hurling praise at me and willing me up the climb. Gingerly, my hands were spinning the wheels and my shoulders were hanging. *I am battered but not finished.*

"Go, John, go!" my sister's voice called out. Then I saw Chris standing with my family screaming encouragement, words that were a foreign language to me, but helpful nonetheless. The finish was within reach; I could almost feel it, clawing for every rotation before I steered myself through it and slouched over under the swarm of my support team.

I had nothing to be ashamed of that day in Providence. It had taken me a little over an hour and a half to complete the 13.1-mile run and, overall, seven and a half hours to finish the entire trek. Unlike the ASPIRE 10K where my poor showing demoralized me, now I was filled with the pride of knowing that the course did not beat me that day.

Chris and I had done what we had set out to do, my little turmoil along the way notwithstanding. But nobody ever said that 70.3 miles was going to be a handout. As he congratulated me, he told me his time, five hours fifty minutes, a sub-six hour showing in his first competition. *Now, he's just making me look bad!* We were on the top of the world as we stood on the hill overlooking the city below us and the miles that we had traveled to get there.

26

The red light flashed and a beeping noise announced that our bags would soon be coming off of the conveyer belt. Around it went with the rickety gears grinding with each turn. In my wheelchair waiting for my luggage, I had Dave and Erik by my side. We had just landed from San Diego where Erik had brought Team A Step Ahead to compete in a team triathlon. Like the ASPIRE, it was a friendly competition where we raised money for the Challenged Athletes Foundation (CAF).

The aim of the San Diego Triathlon Challenge, and the CAF as a whole, was to give disabled athletes the opportunity and the inspiration to participate in competition. Furthering the initiative was the money raised, providing disabled athletes with the training and equipment they needed to lead active lifestyles again. For most, insurance did not cover this luxury. While I was able to make it back because of the selfless support that I had received, many others did not receive the same assistance.

Bluntly and unannounced, Erik spouted, "When are you going to run the fuckin' marathon?" We all laughed, but his question was pointed with purpose. It was not a joke; he was as serious as a stroke.

I left Erik and Dave in the airport that day with a maybe, but I still needed to convince myself that I could do it. The New York City Marathon was not a 5K, a 10K, or even a half ironman. It was 26.2 miles on a running prosthetic that still left my shoulders dragging on the ground and my hands feeling like baseball mitts.

Besides, the race was more than a year away; the only competition I was concerned with at that point was the ASPIRE. I still had to prove to myself that I was not the same kid who got lost in the woods and crossed the finish line when nobody was there to see it. When I thought about the

ASPIRE, familiar feelings of failure and disappointment returned to me. They would remain until I did what I was supposed to do the first time.

****

As I came back for my second semester, it dawned upon me that there would be no more after it. This was one of those realizations that was always known but did not truly begin to register until it was about to happen. While some of my classmates already had jobs lined up, I, like many of my peers, faced an uncertain future. I was just beginning to study for my MCAT to at least give myself the option of attending medical school, but I was not sure if I wanted to go right back to school, foster my career as a motivational speaker, or pursue another occupation.

****

When the shores stopped washing up slushy snow, I started to train in the walking leg. The walks, though, would only get me so far in my attempt to compete in the 6.2-mile ASPIRE. For my stamina to reach my ambitions, I had to get into the running prosthetic and go for a run on my own.

Until senior year, I had always been dependent on a partner being alongside me, a precaution in case I fell or needed a drink. While my friends occasionally joined me and my parents were always eager to help, I recognized that it was an inconvenience for them to walk with me for hours. So by the end of February, I devised a way to hydrate while running.

With my car parked in a central location relative to my run, I would set some sports drinks on the roof of my car; this way, I could return for a drink when I needed it but did not have to rely on bringing someone along with me. The questions I had to answer in order to do everyday, functional activities were sometimes astounding, but I made it work and could at least run on my own now.

When that April day finally arrived, I was back at Madeline Middle School in Plainview, Long Island. Yet it was neither friendly nor blithe. This time, I had come prepared to run the race that I should have run last year. This time, I wanted to do *bad things* to that race.

Hitting the course, I was flooded with memories of my past anguish and personal defeat, and I used them as incentive to push myself harder. As I pounded the foot into the ground and jumped into my stride, I still felt the road running up through my arms and into my shoulders, but I was hardened to it; it would not slow me down.

The fences changed from modern to rustic, the houses grew farther and farther apart, and I actually made the right turn this time. Through the business district, I could see the most challenging climb ahead. Busting up the hill with the same strength I had at the beginning of the race and with the crowd cheering me on, I cruised toward the finish line.

As the emcee announced my name, I reveled in the moment. Although I had technically become the first person with no legs to complete a 10K at last year's ASPIRE, the second attempt was the true feat. There were no regrets when I crossed the plane and saw a time of two hours and fifteen minutes. A year later, I was vindicated, doing what I had initially set out to do and shedding the shame of the past in the process. This was the ending that I had imagined last year; now, it was happening.

In the eyes of most, just my completing it, whether it took me two hours or ten hours, was still a sizeable accomplishment. However, I would never settle for the expectations of others.

27

"I want to do it," I said with halfhearted conviction. "I'm young enough, I'm in the best shape of my life, and I don't think I'll ever have this much free time again." For a moment, I had even convinced myself before I began to once again dwell on my doubts. "But I don't know."

Looking for some guidance, some advice, and maybe even some approval, I was unsure if my body could endure the physical trauma of 26.2 miles in the running prosthetic. I would have to train harder than I ever had before. *Is this really what I want to do?*

Brett, with his hand hanging from the steering wheel, glanced over at me through his sunglasses. "You HAVE TO do this," he said unwaveringly.

Since I had completed the hand cycle marathon two years ago, it had been a thought, tucked behind accolades that had to come first. One by one, they had all fallen, checked off the list that was constantly being rewritten. Now, that same urge that had driven me to topple all of the previous competitions was calling on me again. If I could do this, then I could do anything.

There were no longer questions about *if* I could; it was only a matter of when. My mind was set on that first Sunday in November. I would be the first bilateral hip disarticulate to run a marathon—the New York City Marathon.

Erik was as supportive as he was inventive once I told him about my plan to run the marathon. Developing a new S-curve for the second generation running leg, he felt that the design would alleviate pressure on my shoulders and hands while still allowing me to sustain a consistent pace. And it did—at least momentarily.

Running along Fairfield Beach Road had never felt more comfortable. With more of the curve rolling off the ground, the foot leaped from the sanded pavement. My balance instantly leveled too, and I did not even hunch forward when I ran anymore.

Yet the miles I was running those first few days in the newly redesigned running leg were only a microcosm of the training that the future held. I had never come close to stringing together miles like I would have to for the marathon. Even though I would not be running the entire distance of the race straight through in preparing myself for it, I needed to approach the number—in theory, this would allow me to peak during the race as opposed to burning out before I even made it to New York City.

Beyond just a carbon-fiber extension that I strapped to myself, that prosthetic needed to be so broken in that it became as comfortable as my own skin. This took time, though, something I did not have as I attempted to juggle studying for the MCAT and my finals with running. Even if I kept pace with the thirty minutes it took me to run a mile over the 26.2-mile trek, I would finish in approximately thirteen hours.

****

A few weeks before graduation, I received a call from the producers of *Oprah*. They wanted to follow-up on my progress in the years since I had first been featured. I was happy to share how well things were going and what my future plans were. When I Skyped in later that April, Oprah and I chatted about all that had taken place over the past four years– the training, the competitions, the speaking, the college experience. That was all expected. Then came the revelation: I would be running the New York City Marathon. Sharing my secret with viewers across the country made it certain that there was no turning back now. Not that I would have anyway.

Classes stopped, and for some so did the world. Many students did not know what to do. It was the happiest, most depressing time of their lives. They celebrated their graduation with consecutive forgotten nights. And there I was, in the library doing MCAT practice tests. This was what I had come to Fairfield to do as a premed biology major. While I was undecided on when exactly I would attend medical school, I wanted to at least have the option to pursue it.

In high school, I was motivated by my desire to walk to accept my high school diploma. That was not a question now. I had always known that this day would come, that I would walk to the base of the stage and accept my degree under my own power. When my name was called, I stood up from my wheelchair and the crowd stood with me. They were supporting me, befriending me, and making me feel at home like they always had. I took in the scene for a second and raised my crutch in the air to say thank you to everyone behind me. They were cheering for me for who I was, not for what I was doing.

Giada de Laurentiis flashed across the screen. Why she was on the television at the Stonebridge Restaurant where Mike worked over the summer I did not know; however, when the bouncer instructed a gorgeous blonde with lush green eyes and her friend to sit next to me and my friends, I was not complaining. The more I subtly glanced over, the more it became evident that I was interested in her. With a push from Giada, I saw an opportunity.

Intentionally loud, I started to talk about a recent dish I cooked a night ago. "Yeah, that [Giada's pasta] looks good, but it has nothing on the stuffed chicken breast and risotto I just made."

"You a fan of Giada?" I turned toward her. *Contact.*

153

"Not really," she said, not disinterestedly. "I hate the way she pronounces Italian words." As "Par-me-jano" blared from the TV, we both laughed. *Perfect timing, Giada.*

What started as furtive looks and deferential smiles evolved into a lighthearted, then engaging conversation. Her name was Genevieve, and she was from Oxford, Connecticut. We started to learn more about each other—what our interests were, what we wanted to do in the future, and how our days were going so far. Her story was much more interesting than my meeting up with friends from college. She had just escaped a nightmare blind date. She needed to leave her date so she could "tend to an emergency to help her friend." What she really did was drive away and pick up ice cream for the bouncer who promised to save her parking spot.

After laughing together, getting to know each other, and having her open up to me about being on a date before, I knew this had the potential to be something different. This had substance.

Then, the moment of truth came, the rites of passage for all men when meeting a girl for the first time, the validation for if they actually were as smooth as they thought they were.

While I could have said, "So can I have your number?" I really said, "So are you going to give me a kiss or what?"

Laughing, she gave me a kiss along with her number. It felt right. It was right.

Genevieve and I talked again. And again. Through our chance meeting, we became an item—something I could not have expected, walking into the bar to see old friends and walking out with the most important number anyone had ever given me. It had been a couple years since I had had a serious relationship. I had never intended to stay out until eleven having been there since the afternoon, but I was happy that I did. She would change my life. Forever.

Getting my revenge on the 10K after a poor performance the previous year helped me not only to rebuild my confidence but to also spur it forward. I had a lot to prove to myself and to others. This time I didn't train for it; I attacked it. I didn't want to be remembered as the kid who complained throughout the 10K race because he got lost.

Achieving my initial objective made me realize that running a marathon was possible. When pursuing any goal, you have to be able to look at what actions you are taking and be truthful to yourself. Did you really put in the work necessary to achieve your desired outcome?

Understand that no one is perfect and there will always be times where you question yourself; even the most confident do it. But I moved past those fears and took ownership of my performance, and it validated what I knew about myself—that I could do anything when I truly wanted it.

28

Going into Central Park on June 28, I felt confident. Team A Step Ahead events were generally low-pressure competitions, and, besides, I had just done the 6.2-mile ASPIRE a couple of months ago. Sure, I was racing in the modified running leg for the first time, but it was only five miles. This was my chance to show Erik that I was ready for the rigorous road ahead. Unfortunately, the heat clung to me like reigns. And I had forgotten about all of those hills.

Two hours felt like seven as I took agonizing step after agonizing step. Worse, catching a breeze was impossible. Rippling heat waves seemed to blur time until it stopped and I was simply running in place. I might have been one of the youngest competitors there, but on that day I was an old man. Like a punch-drunk prizefighter, I staggered through the finish line.

While I had thought I would be faster in the new prosthetics, in Central Park it took me longer to complete the five miles than my previous 10K. The elevated temperature was clearly an issue, but that was never and would never be an excuse. Searching for a solution, a few weeks after the event I went to Hicksville to see if Erik could modify the running leg to make me move faster. I was training harder than I did for the ASPIRE, so there was no reason for my lagging in Central Park. While he changed the angle from the socket to the foot, he made it clear to me that if I wanted to save my shoulders from the ruin of the road, I would have to give up some speed.

I had gone into the event carefree and without a concern for the course or the distance. But instead of devouring the five miles as an appetizer to the marathon, I panted through Central Park like a tired dog.

Erik, as a friend, questioned my dedication. He had every right to. "I don't want you to get out there if you don't want to do this," he said, "but if you're going to do this, it's going to be a big deal. You NEED to finish."

I had grappled with the question for almost a year. If I cowered at the possibility of failure, I might never have this chance again. I had confronted odds far more bleak than my chances in the marathon and I had persevered. I would again.

"I'm in," I said with brevity that made my decision seem like an easy one.

As the summer seared me through July, I regularly visited the track with one of my parents. Dave was keeping me on a running schedule that built up to the weekend where I would have my most strenuous day of training. Whereas Monday would consist of a two- to four-mile run, by Saturday I would run anywhere from ten to sixteen miles depending on what I had done throughout the week.

While I was not setting the streets ablaze with my blistering speed, I was seeing progress. Yet at the same time, I was struggling with my hands. They were breaking down. My unruly sweat created a constant friction that left them looking and feeling like beef jerky. I had to do something, but whether I adjusted the crutch height or put antiperspirant on my palms, nothing seemed to work. Trying to train through the pain, I found it to be unbearable when the tension began to move into my wrists. Without any other choice, I bought a set of titanium crutches that promised to limit the impact of the ground. Hopefully, they would absorb the shock of the road and mitigate the pain that was wracking my wrists.

****

What I was attempting to do not only had never been done before, but it really did defy reason. This type of competition was not a

158

regular occurrence; it was going to be a fight, and, like any bout, I would need to recover afterward. I was building myself up to compete in an event that would damage me.

"You know, John," my father said as I ran around the block from my house one day, "it's OK if you want to use the hand cycle in the marathon."

There was no discussion to be had. I was adamant in my plans to proceed with training for the marathon, even if it was a slower and more painstaking process in the new running leg.

"There is no challenge to that!" I snapped. "[On *Oprah*] I told the world I was going to do this; there is NO WAY that I'm going to back out now." It was a tumultuous couple of months leading up to the race. He probably thought I was crazy, but I could not settle for what I had already done. I needed to bring out the best in myself.

****

Training had become a full-time job. Logically, as my endurance increased, the hours I spent on the road increased as well; however, in comparison to an able-bodied endurance athlete, it took me longer to run the same distance. While I typically ran a thirty-minute mile, an average, able-bodied male my age generally ran it in about eight minutes.

In the process of running, I expelled more energy than a conventional runner, so race nutrition became a necessary concern of mine. Whereas athletes should consume at least eighteen hundred calories per day, I was taking in between twenty-five hundred and three thousand calories. Even with substantial, protein-laden breakfasts and dinners, it was difficult to recoup the calories that I lost throughout the day.

Since I needed to maintain stamina but could not eat during a run, Gatorades and GU energy supplements took the place of lunch. Initially, my stomach disagreed with the arrangement. The pangs I felt were sometimes as substantive as an actual meal. Hours would pass without any natural sustenance, and the emptiness became analogous with the run. Eventually, I did not feel hunger on the road. I did not even think about it.

My miles were steadily increasing and so too was my confidence. Training on the hilly roads around my house to prepare for the treacherous hikes I would find running in New York City, I felt comfortable enough to try Central Park again. So in early August, I met Dave to atone for my previous misstep.

There, the heat again challenged me as it had earlier in the summer. I breathed out humid flames and felt like I was engulfed in the summer sun. My all-encompassing nemesis threatened to suffocate me, and I knew I could no longer avoid it.

"You have to be ready for any condition," Dave told me as he walked alongside me. "What if it's really hot and muggy out the day of the marathon?"

He was right; I could not use the heat as a crutch for why I did not perform. It did make my trek that much more strenuous, but I could not rest on excuses. The reality was that it would be an utter failure if I did not complete the marathon, regardless of the reason. So we worked for about five hours, covering nine miles of terrain that tested my strength as well as my stamina. Dave even made me go up and down the same hill three times before we continued on in the park. It was tiring and no doubt tedious, but it was what I needed. When I ran the marathon, he would be by my side just as he always was during my races.

Back at home, I hit the track, hit the streets, hit the back roads, hit the beach, hit anywhere that I could put in the miles that would stretch my endurance. There was never a point where I could lean back and say, "Wednesday, I did six miles, so I can skip Friday." I would put forth my best effort in the marathon because pride shows in the work that you do, in the care that you give, and in the struggle that you are willing to overcome. I was going to New York City to run 26.2 miles, and I would not leave until I was done.

Once I began training on the new running leg and putting in the hours necessary to finish the marathon, I started to see what I had gotten myself into. So many of the same problems I had dealt with in the past reemerged all at once. My hands were being eaten up by the crutches and the hours spent on the road. The prosthetic itself was working over my body as it did when I first put it on. Even when I was training, there were issues. I had to find people to walk with me step by step in case I fell or I needed a drink. It just was not practical, and, besides, I didn't want to rely on other people.

What I had been through—losing my legs and coming back from it—had prepared me for the struggle I was going through. While I would get frustrated with my performance at times, I needed to let it go and try again the next day. Sitting up had challenged my morale, my belief in myself, much in the same way this training was. The pain was something I could tolerate. I had felt it before, and worse. Eventually, my body would adjust and it would pass like my back pain did once it became acclimated to the hand cycle.

At the same time, change is disconcerting. It makes you uneasy. Everyone is afraid to accept it since going outside of your comfort zone opens you up for failure. That's what this was for me. I was dealing with more hours on the road than I had ever done before. Realizing that my reactions were normal better equipped me to deal with and accept those changes as they came.

Sure, there will be obstacles, and there certainly will be doubts. Everyone encounters these issues when trying to achieve a goal. The harsh reality is that we have to solve them as they come.

Sometimes, it can be overwhelming to think about the big picture, which leads to further self-doubt. We can control this by taking it one step at a time and knowing that in the next second, minute, hour, or day we have an opportunity to improve our situation. It's about having the right perspective; we have to prepare our minds to accept things we cannot change and make changes to our actions and behaviors when they hinder our progress.

29

The lobby of the Hilton was a Times Square traffic jam of runners. *I can still hear the howls of the crowd in my head.* I had not dreamt about the glory of the marathon the previous night; instead, I had listened to the drunken ghouls of Halloween night in New York City.

With smoke billowing from grates and people's mouths alike and street lamps shining overhead, there was little evidence that the previous night had changed to a new day. Cars were still in garages, taxis did not honk, and vendors had not even dropped off their carts yet. The city that had kept me up all night had conveniently conked out just as I was about to begin my day.

At a little after five, Amy and I hailed a cab. She, my race coordinator and fellow Team A Step Ahead member, was my adopted mother that day. During the marathon, she would monitor my nutrition to make sure that I had enough energy to finish. We would be meeting my parents, Dave, and Richard (a marathon race volunteer) at the start.

Sitting in the backseat with my headphones on and the music blaring, I was trying to pump myself up, but no music could have motivated me more than myself that morning. In the past, I had achieved feats that nobody else with my disability ever had. While I didn't think too much of it, what I was about to do was profound from an "able-bodied" perspective, and, for someone in my position, it was seemingly impossible. However, labels would never define my limits; disabled or not, the New York City Marathon would fall when I crossed the finish line.

It had rained sometime before I made it outside that morning, and the sun was depressed in the overcast sky. A fog was beginning to rise off of the water, and morning was about to break with my race almost underway.

When we first arrived, Dave was waiting for us, as the technicians were just beginning to set up the race. Starting from the same position as the rest of the competitors, I would go off at six, while the push rim racers would start at seven fifteen, the hand cyclists would follow at seven thirty, and, finally, the elite women and men would get going at nine.

Even though I had been there before and I had gone through the course, now, standing three feet higher above the ground, my perspective had changed quite dramatically. For a second, I lost myself in the moment, in the magnitude of the situation. I was not competing in the hand cycle division. I was RUNNING the New York City Marathon. My team of supporters began to surround me as I walked toward the partially set up starting line. This was not a dream. This was as real as waking up one day in the hospital without legs. No gunshot or horn sounded and no crowd cheered. I went on Amy's cue and my time started.

My hands were tightly wrapped around the crutches that slapped against the slippery ground and pushed me onto the Verrazano-Narrows Bridge. I had not noticed it when I had cycled over it three years ago, but the bridge went from cement, to pavement, to metal grates. The first time my crutch hit the grate, I lost traction like a hydroplaning car and almost tasted the cement. I could not let my race end before it started.

Richard, as unfamiliar to me as anyone else on the streets of New York, diligently pushed my wheelchair behind me. He even made little posters with my name on them that he attached to my chair so that when people saw them, they would know who they were cheering for. Ironically, Dave, who had just had ankle surgery, was on crutches next to me. He was the epitome of a racing partner. Amy, along with my parents, rounded out my troop of supporters.

Unlike the last time when I had burned up the streets of New York City in my hand cycle, there were no competitors around me. The road was my only adversary that day. Consumed in the motions of running, I scanned the floor for any imperfections that might throw me off course. While reaching the finish line was still a question, I had a rhythm that was as natural as a street performer slapping a plastic bucket. There was no pain and no pressure, not yet anyway; I was just going, eyes straight ahead, racing against history and myself as well.

My breath was no longer visible in the air. Instead, my body burned with perspiration as steam rose from my radiator chest. Losing a layer of clothing, the air conditioner kicked in and I was back on the beat. But I was not alone out there anymore. The push rimmers zipped past me like high and tight fastballs. I, on the other hand, was going along at a change-up pace.

It had to be a little bit after 9:00 a.m. when the elite women runners began to leave me behind as well. Their strides looked so effortless yet, at the same time, so controlled. I really was only looking at their feet; the scenery was lost upon me during most of the race because my sole focus was on what was directly in front of me. They were moving, faster and faster, until they were simply dots in the distance.

What once was the city and me was now me in the city. I was swallowed up in a sea of people, churning around me and chugging past me. Runners gave their regards, offering me encouragement and calling out my name as they saw it on the back of my wheelchair. Crowds lined the sidewalks, bending the guardrails and bleeding emotion onto the street. I fed off of their unbridled enthusiasm; not that I was tired, but I had been up for as long as Father Time and it was uplifting to have strangers scream your name until they were hoarse. Music was blaring from corner to corner, bases beat against the ground, and my ears were

165

twitching to the thump of guitar chords and inaudible words. Ethnic dishes filled the air with the aromas that announced the passing neighborhoods.

In the commotion of all that was going on, I had forgotten that Amy had set up an in-race interview for me with NBC. At first, I was hesitant to embrace it because I was running a race. The last thing that I wanted was to come off sounding like an idiot on national television. While I secretly hoped that the reporter would not catch up to me, around mile thirteen the microphone was in front of my face and the camera was rolling. The newswoman introduced me, telling the world who I was and how much I had overcome to compete in the marathon. It was the same old story, and I was happy that I did not have to tell it again.

"How are your arms feeling?" she asked.

My words were labored under the strain of my steps. "I'm feeling really strong." With the crowd bellowing from behind, she asked me what cause I was running for.

"I'm out here raising money for ASPIRE, a group that helps youth amputees have the opportunity to participate in athletics," I said as I alternated my glance between the ground and the camera.

"Is there anything that you want to say to the viewers at home?" she said, getting ready to wrap up the spot and move on to the next piece.

"There are no limits to what you can do and don't think that you can't accomplish whatever you want," I said, looking into the lens. "I want to thank everyone who has supported me over the years. Milford, Connecticut, this one goes out to you!"

The red light of the camera flickered out; she wished me luck and then drove off to her next stop.

All the while, the crowd continued to chant and hail the runners as their heroes. For twenty minutes straight, it seemed, there was no pause to their ovation. It only continued to grow until I could feel it beating louder than my heart. I felt like the star baseball player going out for a curtain call after he just hit a clutch home run. Between the energetic audience and the background music that grew more present after each block, I could have confused the scene for a concert if I wasn't running a marathon.

"The best part about this race is that I know I'm going to finish it," I said to my team.

Amy chuckled at my boast. "Even if you couldn't finish it, we would make you!" Richard, meanwhile, was inciting the crowd in my favor. I could hear my name, and it further motivated me to keep moving.

As the runners who were passing me began to thin out, my supporters did not. Sporadically, friends from Fairfield were popping up in the crowd to support to me. They had made the trip to the city; they were there to cheer me on. Around mile sixteen, Brett, my training partner and the guy who had helped me make this decision, joined me on the road. Having him in my stable of supporters really kept me pushing on.

"Your faux hawk is in full force," he said, referring to my hair. Smiling under the strain of my task, I huffed out a laugh. "You look a helluva lot better than I would after all these miles."

The last of the runners made their way around me, dragging themselves past, and I had the streets all to myself again. Even the crowd, which was once as loud as a ballpark, was now a small amphitheater squeaking out support. However, Amy had a surprise for me. As dusk began to settle in and the race was wrapping up, I was floored by the shrieking applause of little children, some from Team A Step Ahead and some from other programs that she worked with. Seeing all of those cute, impressionable youths, some in their prosthetics, clapping and waving at me was awe-inspiring. They were there for me, the thought repeated in my mind, as the gesture took me aback and reminded me of all the support I had had along the way; maybe one day, they too would run the marathon.

With all of the runners having made it through the finish, the race began to close down. I could not expect the marathon to wait for me with roughly thirty thousand participants, but I was still one of those participants. Fortunately, the New York Police Department recognized that my race had not ended. Officers actually kept streets closed longer than they were supposed to just so I would have the chance to finish the race.

It was around 6:00 p.m., and night was beginning to descend; street lamps were lit and headlights were turned on. My breath had returned to the front of my face, and the chill air iced my nose. We were going up First Avenue toward the Willis Avenue Bridge. This was the last bridge I had to cross before I would make my way into Manhattan, through Central Park, and on to the finish. The only problem was that since the race was technically over, the bridge was closed to runners. We could not cross it. With roughly seven miles to go, we had to take a detour that would loop us around the bridge and land us in Central Park where I would be able to officially finish the race.

Unfortunately, this set me back a mile in my already excruciating trek. I was beginning to feel the rigors of the road. While my hands clung to the crutches as if they were cemented on, my shoulders had started to sag and my body strained to support the prosthetics. I tried to block out the emotions of exhaustion, the longing to stop moving, the urge to rest. They would have to wheel me out on a stretcher before I gave up this far into the race.

While I battled through each swing, my eyes remained focused on the ground as the portable iPod set up continued to play Lil Wayne. My team was there for me as they had always been, building me up over the course of my climb. They had even formed a human roadblock so I could keep moving uninhibited by traffic.

"The marathon officials have long gone home," Brett said. "So each of us are going to walk in a line and take up an entire lane of the road [so that John can walk the official path]."

Cars and trucks and buses and cabs drove by, while faces turned and pressed against windows. As their eyes watched the pendulum swing back and forth, time seemed to slow. Their expressions, questioning, wondering, remained stalled in disbelief.

I could see the trees rising up in the distance; we were approaching Central Park. The sidewalks had been quiet for some time now, but as I entered the park, another raucous team of Tartaglio supporters—my sister, my brother-in-law, my girlfriend Genevieve, and my aunt and uncle—joined up with us. I had a smile for Genevieve; she was special. Only a few months into our relationship, I thought we had known each other for years. She knew me, she understood me. Pumped full of encouragement and energy supplements, I continued on into that endless night for her and for the rest of my family.

It had been a long day for everybody. As I fought for each step I was struggling to take, my father started to groan. This persisted for some time with my mother continually shoving him and telling him to "Shut up! Your son is running the marathon!" I was too tired to laugh, but I smiled at their playful fighting. My father, always the emotional one, could never hide his feelings. My mother, on the other hand, was slightly more composed. Regardless, they both would have walked the marathon on broken ankles if that was what was best for our family. Together, they had given me the means to be the person that I always was.

Genevieve, meanwhile, was poker-face reserved for the sake of my focus. Her silent dedication pushed me to keep going; even without her saying it at first, I knew how much she wanted me to finish—for myself, for her, for us. Now, with the night enveloping us, sealing most of the light in the obscure darkness, she held a flashlight shining in front of me the whole time. We were in this together.

However, around the twenty-fourth mile, I hit a wall that came out of nowhere like a stop sign behind a tree. It was then that she knew I needed her the most.

"You can do this," she said with the quiet confidence of someone who believes in you regardless of the circumstance, with the conviction of someone who will never bet against you.

Yet my body crashed with such a sluggish fatigue that it left me paralyzed. Shakily planting my crutches against the ground, I pushed myself forward, but my swing was more like a dripping spit. I became a slow-motion setting until finally I hit pause and leaned against my father to catch my breath. *This is it.*

If only it were that easy. Before I could procrastinate any longer, Dave and Amy were in my ear.

"Come on, John!" They said together. "You have to keep going! Let's go!"

You can do this. Amy gave me a squirt of Gatorade and shoved some cake batter into my mouth. *You can do this.* I had not come this far to quit. *You can do this.* With my team behind me pleading with me, yelling as loudly as crowds I had passed hours earlier, I slowly began to move forward again.

It was not only my team following me, though. A middle-aged man on a bike circled around us, telling us how he was so amazed by what I was doing that he had to get other people to see it for themselves. And he did. There were about fifty people with me. We were like a parade marching down the block and I was the conductor.

All along, there was only one thought in my mind: I would not stop until I crossed that tape. Then, I realized that there would not be any tape, nor would there be anyone awaiting my finish. The race had ended hours ago.

When I saw the twenty-six-mile marker, I knew that, so long as a car did not hit me in the next .2 miles, I was going to make it. I would be mobbed by my closest family and friends, people who had been with me since the beginning, people who had affected me just as much as I had affected them.

Finally, looking up from the ground, the ING banner still hung from the scaffolding that had not been taken down. And in the dark, desolate night against the illuminated backdrop, I could see the outline of red tape strung across the finish line. Even the crowd that I never really thought would be there actually was, their valiant voices leading my way to the finish.

With flashlights shining on me, pulsing cop car lights at my back, and cameras flashing, I dug down into parts of my body that did not even exist anymore and threw myself into each stride like it was a long jump. This was the culmination of all that I had worked for—from the hospital bed, to the rehab facility, back into home life, to my return to high school, to the moment I accepted my diploma, all I had ever wanted was to be like the next guy. Now, I was doing him one better. I was about to complete the New York City Marathon.

As the tape fell like a pristine ribbon in the wind, I stopped at the line and did not cross through it. Exhaling the deepest breath of my entire life and with tears in my eyes, I held my arms up like a champion and eased myself back into my mother—my strength—who wrapped her arms around my torso. As the camera bulbs snapped at a seizing clip, one of the remaining race workers draped a medal around my neck. I had done what no one else before me had ever done. And while I considered myself as normal as the next kid, what I had done simply was not. I had dared to dream of a life that exceeded being wheelchair bound and dependent on others for survival. This was the surreal, the unbelievable, but it was not the impossible.

"Come forward," the race workers said. They wanted me to cross the finish line.

I simply shook my head. "Na, I'm done." I had made it, and I would not go one step farther.

With their faces skewed by the shadows cast across them, people shouted me praise through the blind night. Smothered in backslaps, kisses, and hugs, I collapsed into the backseat of a golf cart that would bring us back to our car. And there was Genevieve. She had seen my pain, my struggle, had worried about me, had pulled for me; she couldn't imagine what my body was going through. It was hard for her to watch, but she walked with me the whole night because she knew how much completing the marathon meant to me.

When I rested against her, I could hear the pride in her voice as she lauded me with words, love, and a kiss. We went around in the cart to see all those people who had stayed until ten at night to witness my almost sixteen-hour journey. My official time for completing the New York City Marathon was exactly 15 hours, 59 minutes, and 59 seconds, but the number didn't matter. The accomplishment did, and nobody could ever take that away from me.

While it was tragic that at seventeen, I had lost my legs and my left bicep to a bacterium that gave no reason for its choice, what really would have been heartbreaking was if I had decided to give up. I had made it back from a place that most do not because I was able to find closure in a situation that had none. There was no reasoning with what had happened to me, and I could not fight fate. So I attacked my disability instead and, in the struggle, discovered that there was more to life than legs.

The miracle of my story was not that I had survived, but instead that I had continued to thrive in college, in competition, in leading the life that I had always intended to live. For as much as I had lost on August 22, 2004, and as crazy as Spellman thought that I was at first, I still considered myself lucky. If I still had my legs, I never would have gotten in the pool, or signed up for a triathlon, or competed in a half ironman. There would have been no Jim, no Erik, no Spellman, no Amy, not even Richard. No ASPIRE, no 5K benefit, and no Jog-A-Thon at Royal Middle School. Who knows if I would have gone to Fairfield U to stay close to home; then, I never would have met friends at the restaurant, which means I never would have met Genevieve.

My disability did not define me; there was no distinction that could limit my aspirations. What I had been through and what I had overcome was the resistance training of my life. Life had berated me, beaten me down, and pushed as hard as it could to force me into submission. And I had held the line, maintaining my position and never forgetting who I was throughout the whole ordeal.

It was not until I rested against my mother's chest that I felt the weight of the world shift from my shoulders. I breathed out years' worth

173

of toil and realized that marathon moment as a triumph that I could hold my head up to. All of the other accolades that I had accomplished were recognized as astounding, remarkable, unfathomable, but they were never that to me. They were simply competitions and I was just another competitor. But as the workers began to break down the scaffolding, the police lights flickered out, and the cameras stopped clicking, I embraced the endless night that I had ventured into over four years ago. This was my life, a life that at one point was not guaranteed.

Wrapped in a blanket of praise, I was standing as the only person with no legs to ever complete a marathon, the New York City Marathon. And for the first time, I felt comfortable in it.

EPILOGUE

How did I go from being told that I would never walk again to deciding that I wanted to become the first person with no legs to run a marathon? Well, I like to think that I was the only one dumb enough to give it a shot. Really though, it was a thought that I planted into my mind after the first few road races I completed. I would joke around about running in a marathon with Erik, asking him if he thought I could do it. And every time, Erik was behind me 100 percent because there was part of me that was serious.

Preparing relentlessly day after day outside on the road all led up to November 1, 2009. This was my day to take a stroll through the park with some friends. All of the hours I had endured over the past five and a half months went by so quickly, but that long day will be ingrained in my memory forever.

The feeling of being out on the road running for sixteen hours is scary to most, but it was a day I looked forward to. It was my day to prove to myself that I had what it took to do something that I had never even thought was possible. I was anticipating that great feeling you get when you accomplish a goal you set out to achieve. But this was a different goal; this was an opportunity to do something no one else had ever done.

Seeing the finish line, falling back against my mother, and throwing my arms into the air was the moment that I saw a dream turn into reality. It meant much more to me than accomplishing something that no one else had ever done before. That moment was the best form of gratitude that I could offer to those who cared so much about me. In my mind, this moment cemented the notion that I had persevered through a series of life-changing events that many people tell me they never could have dealt with. To me, it was symbolic; I had undoubtedly overcome my disability.

While I know that I will never be able to give enough credit to those who have helped me, their constant encouragement and praise for my efforts reinforced how critical it is to have those in your life who support you, who impress positive values on you, and who steer you in the right direction. Why does it take a catastrophe to bring people, families in particular, closer together? It shouldn't. Life is too short to distance yourself from the people you care about. Be appreciative of them and empower them to do what you know they are capable of, even if it defies all odds.

And I understand that some may not have the strong family bond that I was blessed with for this type of guidance; however, there are different types of family. Family does not have to be constrained by blood; family is who you surround yourself with.

Think about who you would go to for advice, the people who help you put things into perspective when you are down, the people who will tell you what you need to hear. Because sometimes, your biggest supporters will not be your blood relatives. By surrounding yourself with people who not only believe in you but will also tell you what is in your best interest, this will make you a successful person. If you trust them and believe in yourself and you are dedicated to pursuing what you want, you should be able to look back on your efforts with no regrets.

Everyone has adversity and personal hardships they battle with throughout their lives. I would never think to dismiss or compare someone's situation to my own. No person's problems are too small, and every one of them comes with different backgrounds and life experiences. This book is not intended to make anyone feel bad about complaining. I have been told that after people hear my story, they feel obligated to "never complain again." It is not about that. We are all human, and humans complain by nature. What my adversity is will be different than your adversity, but it doesn't make it any less difficult. This book is intended to help you handle these tough times with a new approach. It is about believing in yourself, challenging yourself to be better, and appreciating who you have around you.

To this day, I continue living my life in a way that means the most to me. I'm proud to say that I found the love of my life in Genevieve Robinson, now Genevieve Tartaglio. We have a beautiful little girl, Lillian Eleanor, who brings so much joy into our lives every day. In the same way I have had to overcome adversity in the past, there are the welcomed struggles of adapting to becoming a new father in the present. Genevieve and I tackle them together, as a team, enjoying each moment and knowing how special it is.

I still travel as a motivational speaker, sharing my journey with audiences. I'm always happy to hear the positive feedback from audience members after I speak as it lets me know I've met my objective of impacting someone's life in a positive way. My mission as a speaker is to ensure that people know that they can achieve anything they want when they pursue what they value and work hard for it.

I continue challenging myself academically and, as a result, am receiving my MBA in 2014. I have always valued education because of the opportunities it will afford me in the future. Ultimately, I want to help businesses diagnose and solve problems to improve their performance.

All of us want to leave a legacy behind in which we are remembered for the impact we have had. In trying to leverage the skills I've learned and the experiences that I've had, I want to affect as many lives as I can for the better.

Each of us has opportunities every day to impact our own lives and the lives of others, so I leave you with a challenge—a challenge to inspire, a challenge to influence, a challenge to make a difference. Remember that people are always watching you, so know that how far you fall does not determine who you are; it's how hard you work to get back up.

ABOUT THE AUTHORS

John Tartaglio is a professional motivational speaker who has traveled across the nation telling his story. His mission is to inspire people to pursue what they value and, in doing so, allow them to see that they can achieve anything they want. Only five years after being told that he would never walk again, in November 2009 John became the first person with no legs ever to run a marathon. John, a 2009 graduate of Fairfield University, will be an MBA graduate from the University of Connecticut in 2014. He loves competing in triathlons, road races, and cycling events and spending time with his wife and daughter along with other family and friends.

Andrew Chapin is a middle school English teacher in New Rochelle, NY, who always dreamed of being a published author. In 2010, John Tartaglio offered him the break he was looking for–a chance to develop a book about John's life, an idea that eventually spawned FROM TRAGEDY TO TRIUMPH. Andrew, who majored in English and graduated from Fairfield University in 2009, recently completed his MS in adolescent English education at Iona College. Recently, he became engaged to the love-of-his-life and moved to Manhattan's Upper East Side. Thankful for the family and friends who have enabled him to pursue his passion, Andrew looks forward to the boundless possibilities that lie ahead.